DIABETIC COOKBOOK FOR THE
NEWLY DIAGNOSED

Maintain Healthy Living with 1800 Days of Easy and Flavorful Recipes - Includes Comprehensive 60-Day Meal Plan and 2 Exclusive Bonuses

By

Susan Elliott

TABLE OF CONTENTS

INTRODUCTION

Chronic diabetes hampers glucose utilization and insulin regulation, resulting in high blood sugar levels and potential health complications. A diabetes diagnosis requires significant lifestyle and dietary changes, which can be overwhelming. To assist newly diagnosed individuals, diabetic cookbooks prove invaluable. These collections of recipes are tailored to manage diabetes through healthy, balanced meals. Typically, they offer low-sugar, low-carb, high-protein, and high-fiber recipes to maintain stable blood sugar levels. Beyond delicious dishes, these cookbooks provide advice on diabetes management, including meal planning, portion control, carbohydrate counting, and selecting nutritious ingredients. They empower individuals to make

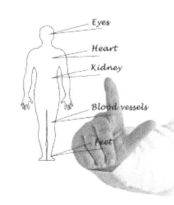

informed decisions about their diet and lifestyle, leading to improved health and well-being. Diabetic cookbooks come in various types, focusing on specific cuisines or dietary needs, and may include meal plans and grocery lists. When choosing a cookbook, personal preferences, dietary requirements, and accurate nutritional information should be considered. Ultimately, a diabetic cookbook plays a crucial role in helping individuals newly diagnosed with diabetes take charge of their health, make informed choices, and effectively manage their condition, ultimately enhancing their overall quality of life.

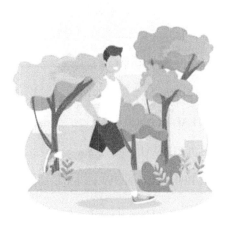

CHAPTER 1: OVERVIEW OF NEWLY DIAGNOSED DIABETES

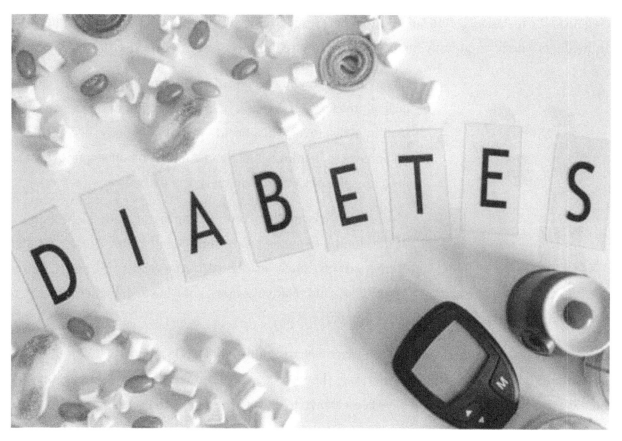

Many people may feel anxious and overwhelmed after learning they have diabetes, especially those who have just received their diagnosis. It's critical to realize that controlling diabetes necessitates ongoing lifestyle adjustments in order to keep one's health in tip-top shape.

Type 1 and type 2 diabetes are the two primary subtypes of the disease. The immune system of the body destroys the insulin-producing cells in the pancreas, resulting in type 1 diabetes. As a result, type 1 diabetics must administer insulin intravenously or employ an insulin pump to control their blood sugar levels. Despite typically first developing in childhood or teenagers, type 1 diabetes can also affect adults.

Type 2 diabetes happens when the body becomes resistant to the effects of insulin or when the pancreas can no longer produce enough insulin to meet the body's needs. Type 2 diabetes is more common than type 1 diabetes and is typically correlated with dietary, physical activity, and weight choices. While type 2 diabetes can be managed with lifestyle changes, some people may additionally need medication or insulin to maintain blood sugar control.

1.1 WHY DO CERTAIN PEOPLE DEVELOP DIABETES

Diabetes can have multiple causes.

Genetics, for instance, is one such factor that can increase the risk of type 1 and type 2 diabetes. Individuals who have a family history of diabetes are more prone to the disease.

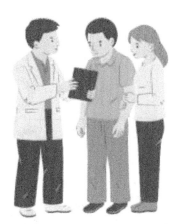

Lifestyle also plays a crucial role, where unhealthy eating habits, lack of physical activity, and being overweight or obese can cause insulin resistance. This occurs when the body becomes less responsive to insulin, which leads to high blood sugar levels and increases the risk of developing type 2 diabetes.

Moreover, age is another contributing factor, with the probability of developing diabetes rising significantly after age 45. Certain ethnic groups, such as African Americans, Hispanic/Latino Americans, and Native Americans, have a higher chance of developing type 2 diabetes than other populations.

Certain medical conditions, such as polycystic ovary syndrome (PCOS), pancreatic disease, and hormonal imbalances, can also increase the risk of developing diabetes. Finally, certain medications like corticosteroids have been shown to elevate the risk of diabetes.

1.2 HOW DO YOU KNOW IF YOU HAVE DIABETES

There are a number of signs and symptoms that diabetes may be present. It's crucial to remember that some diabetics, especially in the beginning stages of the disease, may not even exhibit any symptoms. People who are at risk of getting diabetes should get regular checks for the disease.

Here are a few typical diabetic warning signs and symptoms:

- Frequent urination: One of the earliest indications of diabetes is frequently this. More frequent trips to the bathroom may be the result of the body's attempt to flush off more glucose through the urine.
- Increased urination can also result in dehydration, which can result in excessive thirst.
- Fatigue: The body may find it challenging to convert glucose into energy when blood sugar levels are high, leaving one feeling weak and weary.

- Vision blur: High blood sugar levels can cause fluid to be drawn from the tissues of the eyes, which can result in vision loss.
- Wounds that take a long time to heal: High blood sugar levels can hinder the body's capacity to recover, which can result in infections and wounds that take a long time to heal.
- Tingling or numbness in the hands or feet: Nerve damage brought on by high blood sugar levels can result in tingling, numbness, or pain sensations in the hands and feet.

1.3 COMPLICATIONS ATTRIBUTED TO DIABETES

Numerous short-term and long-term effects can result from diabetes if it is not properly treated. A multitude of health problems may develop over time as a result of excessive blood sugar levels harming the body's blood vessels and organs. Among the most prevalent issues related to diabetes are those listed below:

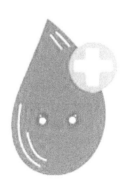

- Cardiovascular disease: which includes conditions like peripheral artery disease, heart attack, and stroke and diabetes both increase the risk of these conditions.
- Harm to the kidneys: Chronic high blood sugar levels can eventually lead to kidney failure due to diabetic nephropathy.
- Eye damage: High blood sugar levels can damage the blood vessels in the eyes, leading to diabetic retinopathy, which can cause vision loss.
- Diabetic neuropathy, which can tingle, numb, or hurt the hands and feet, can be caused by high blood sugar levels damaging the body's nerves.
- Diabetes can cause poor circulation and damage to the nerves in the foot, increasing the risk of injuries and infections.
- Skin problems: Fungal infections, diabetic dermopathy, and other skin problems, such as skin infections, are more common among diabetics.
- Hearing impairment: Hearing loss has been linked to a higher risk of diabetes.

Risk of stroke

Diabetes can increase the risk of stroke due to the effect of high blood sugar levels on blood vessels

Risk of heart disease

Diabetes can increase the risk of heart disease due to the effect of high blood sugar levels on the heart and blood vessels.

Fatigue

Feeling tired and low in energy can be a symptom of high blood sugar levels.

Frequent urination

Due to the increased thirst, people with type 2 diabetes may also experience more frequent urination.

Foot pain or numbess

You may experience numbness or pain in your feet.

Increased thirst

People with type 2 diabetes may experience an increased feeling of thirst as the body tries to compensate for the excess sugar in the bloodstream.

High blood pressure

Diabetes can increase the risk of high blood pressure, which can lead to heart disease and stroke.

Numbness or tingling

You may experience numbness or tingling in your hands.

Dry skin

High blood sugar levels can lead to dry skin and other skin conditions.

1.4 TESTS AND DIAGNOSIS FOR NEWLY DIAGNOSED DIABETES

To diagnose diabetes, healthcare providers may use one or more of the following tests.

- FPG test: This examination assesses your blood sugar level following an overnight fast. (Usually 8 hours). A blood sample is drawn, and the lab receives it for examination. Diabetes is indicated by readings of 126 mg/ld or greater on two different occasions.

- Oral Glucose Tolerance Test (OGTT): This test gauges your blood sugar level following a minimum of an eight-hour fast and a sugary beverage. Over the following few hours, blood samples are obtained at regular intervals to assess your body's capacity to metabolize glucose. After two hours, a value of 200 mg/ld or greater indicates diabetes.

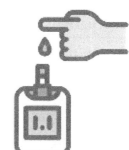

- Tests to determine your average blood sugar levels over the previous two to three months include the hemoglobin A1C (HbA1c) test. When the result is 6.5% or higher, diabetes is suspected.

- Random Plasma Glucose Test: Irrespective of when you last ate, this test analyzes your blood sugar level at any time of day. When combined with diabetic symptoms, a test of 200 mg/ld. or greater suggests the presence of the disease.

1.5 DIABETES TREATMENT

Millions of individuals throughout the world suffer from the chronic disease of diabetes. Despite the fact that diabetes has no known cure, there are a number of treatment choices that can help control the symptoms and enhance quality of life. Some of the most popular diabetes treatments are listed below:

- Alterations in way of life: Making lifestyle adjustments is one of the best methods to manage diabetes. This involves maintaining a healthy weight, exercising frequently, eating a balanced diet, and giving up smoking. You can assist control your blood sugar levels and enhance your general health by making these modifications.

- A number of drugs are available to assist treat diabetes. These include oral drugs that improve how effectively the body uses insulin as well as the hormone insulin, which is used to control blood sugar levels.

- Monitoring your blood sugar levels frequently is essential for good diabetes management. A straightforward blood glucose meter can be used to determine how much glucose is in your blood.

- Insulin pumps: Insulin pumps are machines that continually dispense insulin to the body. With less need for daily injections, persons with diabetes may be able to better control their blood sugar levels.
- Surgery: To assist manage diabetes, surgery may occasionally be advised. This covers operations like gastric bypass surgery, which can assist obese people in losing weight and enhancing their insulin sensitivity.

1.6 DIABETES PREVENTION

In order to preserve excellent health and lower the risk of having this chronic condition, diabetes prevention is essential. The following are some powerful methods for preventing diabetes:

- Keeping a healthy weight in mind: One of the largest risk factors for having diabetes is being overweight or obese. You can considerably lower your risk of having the illness if you maintain a healthy weight through regular exercise and a balanced diet.
- Exercise frequently: Maintaining a healthy weight and boosting insulin sensitivity are two ways that regular exercise can help avoid diabetes. On most days of the week, try to get in at least 30 minutes of moderate exercise, like brisk walking.
- Eat a nutritious diet: By supplying necessary nutrients and assisting in the maintenance of a healthy weight, a diet high in fruits, vegetables, whole grains, lean meats, and healthy fats will help avoid diabetes.
- Avoid sugary drinks: Studies have connected sugary drinks, like soda and fruit juice, to a higher risk of getting diabetes. Instead, choose unsweetened beverages or water.
- Regularly examine your health Regular check-ups with your doctor can help you find the first indications of diabetes and other illnesses, enabling early intervention and treatment.
- Give up smoking: Diabetes and other chronic illnesses are greatly increased by smoking. You can dramatically lower your risk of acquiring diabetes and enhance your general health by giving up smoking.

1.7 MYTHS AND FACTS ABOUT DIABETES

Millions of individuals throughout the world suffer with diabetes, a chronic illness. But numerous diabetes myths and misconceptions might cause misunderstandings and misinformation. Here are some common diabetes myths and realities:

- **Myth: Consuming excessive amounts of sugar leads to diabetes.**

Fact: Although excessive sugar consumption can play a role in type 2 diabetes development, it is not the only contributing factor. Moreover, there are other risk factors at play, including genetics, obesity, and a sedentary lifestyle.

- **Myth: Diabetes is not an acute illness.**

Fact: A number of significant problems, including as heart disease, nerve damage, renal disease, and visual loss, can arise from diabetes. To avoid these consequences, it's crucial to carefully control diabetes.

- **Myth: Sugary foods and carbohydrates are off limits to diabetics.**

Fact: People with diabetes can still occasionally indulge in sweets and carbohydrates. Balanced blood sugar levels can only be achieved through balanced food, frequent exercise, and, if necessary, medication.

- **Myth: Diabetes only affects overweight people.**

Fact: Although being overweight increases the chance of developing diabetes, the disease can also strike the skinny. Diabetes can develop for a variety of reasons, including genetics and lifestyle choices.

- **Myth: Diabetes can be treated with insulin.**

Fact: While used to treat diabetic management, insulin is not a cure-all. For the remainder of their lives, people with diabetes will need to take insulin or other drugs, adjust their lifestyles, and manage their illness.

- **Myth: Diabetics are unable to engage in physical activity.**

Fact: Regular exercise is crucial for controlling diabetes and enhancing general health. Diabetes patients should collaborate with their medical professionals to create a safe and efficient fitness program.

We can better control the condition and lower the risk of complications by grasping the facts about diabetes and busting popular myths. For the best possible health and well-being, it's crucial to collaborate closely with medical professionals and take an active part in controlling diabetes.

CHAPTER 2: DIABETIC DIET

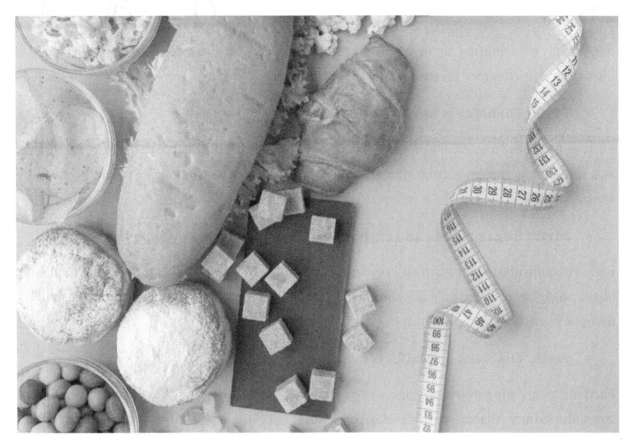

A diabetes diet is a nutritious eating schedule created to help diabetics manage their blood sugar levels. A diabetes diet's major objective is to provide a balanced meal while limiting foods that could quickly raise blood sugar levels. High blood sugar levels can cause a number of health issues, including kidney disease, heart disease, and nerve damage, so understanding this is crucial.

2.1 WHY DO YOU COUNT CARBS?

Counting carbs is a key strategy used by diabetics to manage their blood sugar levels. After a meal, blood sugar levels can be quickly increased by a specific type of nutrition called a carbohydrate. By monitoring the amount of carbohydrates consumed at each meal, people with diabetes can better manage their blood sugar levels and avoid dangerous spikes or drops in blood sugar.

Monitoring the quantity of carbs ingested at each meal and snack is known as carb counting. Reading food labels, using measuring spoons and cups, or utilizing a smartphone app to track carbohydrate intake are all effective ways to accomplish this.

By keeping track of their carbohydrate intake, diabetics can dosage their prescriptions, such as insulin or oral drugs, more precisely and keep their blood sugar levels within a healthy range.

Additionally, it can support people in making educated decisions on the kinds and quantities of food they consume.

While carbohydrate counting is an effective technique for managing diabetes, it is not necessary for all people with the disease. Some people might be able to control their blood sugar levels using different tactics, like portion restriction or adhering to a diet plan that is suitable for those with diabetes.

2.2 GLYCEMIC INDEX: WHAT IS IT?

The glycemic index is a technique used to quantify how quickly and how much a product elevates blood sugar levels after it is consumed. Glycemic index (GI) scores are given to foods based on how they affect blood sugar levels in relation to a reference food, typically glucose or white bread, which has a GI score of 100.

White bread, white rice, and sugary snacks are examples of foods with a high GI score that are quickly digested and induce a sharp increase in blood sugar levels. Contrarily, foods with a low GI score, like whole grains, fruits, and vegetables, digest more slowly and result in a spike in blood sugar levels that happens gradually.

Food's GI score can be influenced by a number of things, such as the kind of carbohydrates it includes, how processed it is, and whether or not it contains fiber, protein, or fat. A food with a high fiber or protein content, for instance, can have a lower GI rating because these nutrients slow down the breakdown and absorption of carbs.

For people with diabetes or other diseases that necessitate constant monitoring of blood sugar levels, the glycemic index can be a helpful tool. People can better control their blood sugar levels and lessen their risk of consequences from high blood sugar by selecting foods with a lower GI score.

2.3 DIABETIC-FRIENDLY FOODS

Foods that are suitable for people with diabetes are those that are high in fiber, have a low glycemic index, and are low in carbohydrates. These foods can aid diabetics in controlling their blood sugar levels and enhancing their general well-being.

Foods that are suitable for people with diabetes include:

- Veggies without grains: Broccoli, spinach, carrots, and peppers are a few of these. They include a lot of fiber, vitamins, and minerals but few carbs.

- Whole grains: Whole grains have a lower glycemic index than processed grains and are higher in fiber. Examples of whole grains are brown rice, quinoa, and whole wheat bread.
- Fish, tofu, and skinless chicken are examples of lean proteins. They make you feel full and satisfied since they are low in carbs.
- Nuts and seeds: Nuts and seeds, including almonds, walnuts, and chia seeds, are rich in fiber and good fats that can aid with blood sugar regulation.
- Dairy goods with low fat: Dairy products with low fat, such yoghurt and cheese, are a good source of calcium and protein. But it's crucial to pick low-sugar options.

2.4 WHICH FOODS TO AVOID AND WHY?

Foods heavy in sugar, saturated fats, and refined carbs should be avoided or consumed in moderation when controlling diabetes since they can elevate blood sugar levels and increase the risk of complications. Among the foods to limit or avoid are:

- Drinks that are heavy in sugar can quickly raise blood sugar levels. Examples include soda, fruit juice, sweetened tea, and coffee.
- Processed snacks: Foods like cookies, crackers, and potato chips are frequently heavy in harmful fats and refined carbs, which can cause weight gain and impair blood sugar regulation.
- Foods that are fried: Foods that are fried, such fried chicken or french fries, are rich in harmful fats and can lead to inflammation in the body, which can exacerbate insulin resistance and raise the risk of problems.
- High-fat meats: Sausage, bacon, and fatty beef cuts are examples of meats that are high in saturated fats and can raise cholesterol levels and increase the risk of heart disease.
- White bread and pasta: White bread and pasta are created from white flour, which has a high glycemic index and can quickly raise blood sugar levels.

2.5 PLANNING A DIET FOR DIABETES

When designing a diet for diabetes, it's important to select foods that are high in fiber, have low glycemic indexes, and are low in carbohydrates. This can assist diabetics in controlling their blood sugar levels and enhancing their general health.

The following actions can be taken to organize a diabetes-friendly diet:

- Choose vegetables without starches: Broccoli, spinach, and carrots are examples of non-starchy vegetables that are strong in fiber, vitamins, and minerals but low in carbohydrates. At every meal, try to fill half of your plate with non-starchy vegetables.

- Choose whole grains: Whole grains have a lower glycemic index than processed grains and are higher in fiber. Some examples of whole grains include brown rice, quinoa, and whole wheat bread. Aim to include whole grains in at least 50% of your grain selections.

- Don't forget lean proteins: Skinless chicken, fish, and tofu are examples of lean proteins that are low in carbs and help you feel full and content. At every meal, try to incorporate a source of lean protein.

- Include healthy fats: Healthy fats, such those in nuts, seeds, avocados, and olive oil, can aid in reducing inflammation in the body and helping to regulate blood sugar. At each meal, try to include a small quantity of healthy fat.

- Sugary and processed foods should be restricted or avoided since they might cause blood sugar levels to surge. Examples of these items include soda, candy, and processed snacks.

- Watch your portions: It's crucial to watch your portions to avoid taking too many carbohydrates at once, which can lead to blood sugar spikes. Your particular needs and goals might help you decide the proper portion sizes by working with a licensed dietitian.

-

2.6 TIPS TO STICK TO YOUR DIET PLAN FOR DIABETES

It can be difficult to follow a diet plan for diabetes, but with the right tactics and pointers, you can succeed. Here are some suggestions to help you follow your diabetes eating plan:

- Set achievable objectives: Achieving achievable objectives will keep you motivated and committed to your diet plan. Start with modest objectives and progress to bigger ones over time.

- Meal planning can help you choose healthier options and prevent impulsive eating. Make a weekly meal plan and try your best to stick to it.

- Maintain a supply of nutritious snacks: Having healthy snacks on hand, such as raw fruit, veggies, or nuts, can prevent you from reaching for unhealthy ones.

- Read food labels: Being able to do so will enable you to make educated decisions about the foods you consume. Pay close attention to the portion sizes and the amount of sugars, fats, and carbohydrates in the food.

- Keep a food journal: A food journal can be used to track your eating patterns and highlight areas that require change. Record everything you consume, then review it frequently to make any necessary improvements.

- Maintain a supply of nutritious snacks: Having healthy snacks on hand, such as raw fruit, veggies, or nuts, can prevent you from reaching for unhealthy ones.

- Read food labels: Being able to do so will enable you to make educated decisions about the foods you consume. Pay close attention to the portion sizes and the amount of sugars, fats, and carbohydrates in the food.

- Keep a food journal: A food journal can be used to track your eating patterns and highlight areas that require change. Record everything you consume, then review it frequently to make any necessary improvements.

- get assistance Having a support network can make it easier to follow your eating plan. Join a support group for people with diabetes, or work with a licensed dietician who specializes in diabetes care.

- Manage your stress: Stress can frequently cause overeating or bad food choices. To handle stress, engage in stress-relieving activities like yoga, meditation, or deep breathing exercises.

CHAPTER 3: DIABETES BREAKFAST

3.1 Scrambled eggs with spinach and raspberry

- o Preparation time: 5 minutes
- o Cooking time: 5 minutes
- o Serving: 1

Ingredients

- o 1 teaspoon canola oil
- o 2 large-size eggs, lightly beaten
- o 1 ½ cups of baby spinach
- o ¼ teaspoon pepper, ground
- o ¼ teaspoon kosher salt
- o ½ cup raspberries
- o 1 slice (whole-grain) bread, toasted

Directions:

- o In a little nonstick skillet, heat the oil over medium-high heat. Add the spinach and simmer for 1 to 2 minutes, frequently stirring, until wilted. Onto a platter, transfer the spinach. Clean the pan, then add eggs and cook it up over medium-low. To guarantee an even cooking, toss the mixture twice during the last minute or two of cooking. Add the spinach, salt, and pepper, and stir. Scramble is best served with bread and raspberries.

Nutritional facts:

- o Calories 296
- o Fat: 15g
- o Carbs: 20g

- o Protein: 21g
- o Sugar: 8g

3.2 Fried veggies and eggs

- o Preparation time: 2 minutes
- o Cooking time: 10 minutes
- o Serving: 1

Ingredients

- o 2 large-size eggs
- o ½ avocado (3½ ounces), wedges, scooped out
- o 1 tablespoon butter
- o ½ cup (½ ounces) of baby spinach
- o 1 tomato (4 ounces), sliced
- o 1 tablespoon whipping cream
- o 1 cup of coffee
- o pepper and salt, to taste

Directions:

- o In a frying pan, melt butter over medium heat.
- o Eggs should be cracked directly into the pan. Fry the eggs on one side only if you want sunny-side-up eggs. After a few minutes, turn the eggs over and cook for an additional minute for over-easy eggs. Simply let the eggs cook for a few extra minutes if you prefer tougher yolks. Add salt and pepper to taste.
- o Serve with fresh-brewed black coffee or tea with cream, baby spinach, tomato, and avocado.

Nutritional facts:

- o Calories 92
- o Fat: 7g

- o Carbs: 0.4g
- o Protein: 6.27g
- o Sugar: 0.38g

3.3 Oatmeal with milk (overnight)

- o Preparation time: 10 minutes
- o Cooking time: 0 minutes
- o Serving: 4

Ingredients

- o 2 cups of rolled oats
- o 2 cups milk, low-fat
- o 1 teaspoon of lemon zest
- o ⅓ cup of pine nuts
- o ½ teaspoon of vanilla extract
- o 2 apricots, chopped
- o 2 tablespoons of agave nectar (Optional)

Directions:

- o In a big bowl, mix oats, milk, vanilla extract, and lemon zest. Cover and chill for eight hours overnight or until the oats have absorbed the milk.
- o Oatmeal should be mixed with apricots and agave nectar.

Nutritional facts:

- o Calories 319
- o Fat: 11g
- o Carbs: 45g
- o Protein: 12g
- o Sugar: 16g

3.4 Greetings, power parfait

- o Preparation time: 5 minutes
- o Cooking time: 0 minutes
- o Serving: 4

Ingredients

- o 1 medium-size banana
- o 2 1/2 cups strawberries, quartered
- o 2 cups vanilla- yogurt, fat-free (divided use)
- o 1 teaspoon cinnamon, ground (optional)
- o 1/2 cup grape-nut cereal, preferably with almonds and raisins

Directions:

- o Blend the banana until smooth with the yogurt, 1 cup, and cinnamon (if using). Pour into 4 parfait or wine glasses.
- o Each parfait should have a cup of strawberries on top.

Nutritional facts:

- o Calories 142
- o Fat: 8g
- o Carbs: 30g
- o Protein: 6g
- o Sugar: 15g

3.5 Yogurt pancakes

- o Preparation time: 10 minutes
- o Cooking time: 20 minutes
- o Serving: 1 dozen

Ingredients

- o 2 cups of all-purpose flour
- o 1 teaspoon of baking soda
- o 2 tablespoons of sugar

- ¼ cup water
- 2 teaspoons of baking powder
- 2 cups of plain yogurt
- 2 large-size eggs, lightly beaten
- Dried cranberries, coarsely chopped pecans, semisweet chocolate chips, and sliced ripe bananas (optional)

Directions:

- Put the sugar, flour, baking soda, and baking powder in a bowl and stir to mix. Whisk the eggs, yogurt, and water in a separate bowl. Mix dry ingredients just enough to moisten them.
- Pour 1/4 cup portions of batter onto a heated griddle covered in frying spray. Adding optional components is optional. When bubbles appear on top, flip the food and cook until the other side is golden brown.

Nutritional facts:

- Calories 242
- Fat: 5g
- Carbs: 40g
- Protein: 9g
- Sugar: 8g

3.6 Rapidly cooked oats

- Preparation time: 5 minutes
- Cooking time: 5 minutes
- Serving: 1

Ingredients

- ½ cup oats, quick-cooking
- ¼ teaspoon of salt
- 1-ounce milk, low-fat for serving

- 1/8 teaspoon of cinnamon
- 1 cup water / milk, low-fat
- 1 - 2 teaspoons honey, brown sugar or cane sugar for serving

Directions:

- On the stove, combine salt, water (or milk), and a small saucepan up to a boil. Oats are added once the heat is reduced to medium, and they are cooked for 1 minute. Turn off the heat, cover the pan, and let it stand for two to three minutes.
- For microwave: Salt, water (or milk), and oats should all be combined in a 2-cup bowl that is microwave-safe. Use the microwave for 1- 2 minutes on High. Before serving, stir.
- Serve with your preferred garnishes, including milk, sugar, cinnamon, dried fruit, and nuts.

Nutritional facts:

- Calories 150
- Fat: 3g
- Carbs: 27g
- Protein: 5g
- Sugar: 1g

3.7 Breakfast bowl with quinoa

- Preparation time: 5 minutes
- Cooking time: 15 minutes
- Serving: 1

Ingredients

- 2 cups coconut milk
- 1 cup of quinoa, rinsed

- Vanilla Greek yogurt, Ground cinnamon sugar substitute blend, honey, fresh blueberries, brown sugar, raisins, chia seeds, chopped apple, and fresh mint leaves (optional)

Directions:

- Milk should be heated to a boil in a big pot while occasionally stirring. The quinoa. Reduce heat; simmer for 12 to 15 minutes with the lid on. With a fork, remove from the heat. Add any assortment of alternative ingredients if desired.

Nutritional facts:

- Calories 217
- Fat: 5g
- Carbs: 33g
- Protein: 10g
- Sugar: 6g

3.8 Mushroom-cheese omelet

- Preparation time: 4 minutes
- Cooking time: 6 minutes
- Serving: 2

Ingredients

- 6 ounces mushrooms, sliced
- 1/8 teaspoon of black pepper
- 1/8 teaspoon of salt
- 1/3 cup green onion, finely chopped
- 1-ounce bleu cheese, crumbled
- 1 cup of egg substitute
- 1/4 cup (reduced-fat) cheddar cheese, shredded

Directions:

- Heat a little skillet over medium-high heat. Add salt and pepper after coating with nonstick frying spray, and add the mushrooms. Apply nonstick frying spray to the mushrooms and cook for 4 minutes or until tender, stirring constantly.
- After adding the onions, simmer for another minute. The pan to one side.
- Another small skillet should be heated up over medium heat. Spray nonstick cooking spray on the surface, then add the egg substitute. Cook without stirring for one minute. Lift the edges with a rubber spatula to let the undercooked portion run under. Cook for a further 1 to 2 minutes or until the eggs are almost set and puffing slightly.
- Place the mushroom mixture in the center of 1/2 of the omelet, top with cheese, and carefully fold over. To serve, divide in half.

Nutritional facts:

- Calories 137
- Fat: 4g
- Carbs: 8g
- Protein: 17g
- Sugar: 3g

3.9 Grilled rye and Swiss cheese

- Preparation time: 4 minutes
- Cooking time: 7 minutes
- Serving: 2

Ingredients

- 4 rye bread slices
- 1/2 cup of egg substitute

- 4 teaspoons (reduced-fat) margarine
- 4 1/2 ounces (reduced-fat) Swiss cheese, sliced

Directions:

- Spread one side of each bread slice with 1 teaspoon of margarine and set aside.

- A medium skillet should be heated up over medium heat. Spray nonstick cooking spray on the surface, then add the egg substitute. Cook without stirring for one minute. Lift the edges with a rubber spatula to let the undercooked portion run under. Cook for a further 1-2 minutes or until the eggs are nearly set and puffing up slightly. 30-second cooking after a flip.

- Half of the eggs should be placed on the unbuttered-sides of two slices of bread after the skillet has been taken from the heat. Place an equal quantity of cheese on each slice of bread, then place the remaining buttered bread slices on top, the buttered side facing down.

- Once more, heat the skillet over medium-high heat. Spray some nonstick cooking spray on the skillet. Cook the two sandwiches for 3 minutes, flip them over and cook for an additional 2 minutes or till golden brown. Each sandwich should be divided in half using a sharp knife.

Nutritional facts:

- Calories 247
- Fat: 8g
- Carbs: 26g

- Protein: 17g
- Sugar: 1g

3.10 Raisins toast with apricot spread

- Preparation time: 8 minutes
- Cooking time: 6 minutes
- Serving: 4

Ingredients

- 8 cinnamon-raisin bread slices
- 1/4 cup of apricot spread
- 3 tablespoons margarine, reduced-fat
- 1 cup of egg substitute, divided use

Directions:

- Place four slices of bread in a 13 x 9-inch baking pan. Spread out 1/2 cup of the egg

  substitute equally, then give everything a few turns to coat. Give the egg two minutes to soak gradually.

- Margarine and fruit spread are mixed thoroughly in a small bowl using a fork in the meantime.

- Heat up a sizable non—stick skillet over moderate heat. Apply nonstick frying spray liberally to the skillet, add 4 slices of bread, and cook for 3 minutes, reserving any leftover egg mixture for the baking pan.

- The bread should be golden brown after 3 more minutes of turning and cooking. Slices should be turned again and cooked for an additional minute for darker toast. Positioned on a serving dish; covered to maintain warmth.

o Place the other slices of bread in the baking dish and evenly distribute the residual egg substitute over everything while the initial batch of them bakes. To coat, rotate many times. Cook as instructed.

o Serve every toast piece.

Nutritional facts:

o Calories 246

o Fat: 6g

o Carbs: 38g

o Protein: 16g

o Sugar: 10g

3.11 French toast

o Preparation time: 15 minutes

o Cooking time: 5 minutes

o Serving: 6

Ingredients

o 4 large-size eggs

o 1 tablespoon of honey

o 1 cup (2%) milk

o 1/2 teaspoon cinnamon, ground

o 12 whole-wheat bread slices

o 1/8 teaspoon of pepper

o vanilla frosting or cinnamon sugar (optional)

Directions:

o Whisk together the eggs, milk, honey, cinnamon, and pepper in a small basin. Dip the bread in the egg mixture on both sides. Cook for 3 to 4

minutes per side on a hot, greased griddle or till golden brown.

o If desired, top with vanilla icing or a cinnamon sugar coating.

Nutritional facts:

o Calories 218

o Fat: 6g

o Carbs: 28g

o Protein: 13g

o Sugar: 8g

3.12 Traditional avocado toast

o Preparation time: 5 minutes

o Cooking time: 0 minutes

o Serving: 1

Ingredients

o 1 hearty bread slice, toasted

o ¼ medium avocado, sliced

o 1 - 2 teaspoons olive oil, extra virgin

o 1/8 teaspoon of sea salt

Directions:

o Olive oil on bread, then avocado slices on top. If preferred, lightly mash the avocado and add more oil. Add a little salt.

Nutritional facts:

o Calories 160

o Fat: 11g

o Carbs: 15g

o Protein: 3g

o Sugar: 1g

3.13 Greek yogurt with nuts and fruits

- o Preparation time: 5 minutes
- o Cooking time: 0 minutes
- o Serving: 1

Ingredients

- o 3 apricots, dried and roughly chopped
- o 1 ½ teaspoons walnuts, chopped
- o ⅓ cup Greek yogurt, nonfat

Directions:

- o In a bowl, put the yogurt. Add the apricots, then top with the walnuts.

Nutritional facts:

- o Calories 93
- o Fat: 2.7g
- o Carbs: 10g
- o Protein: 8.5g
- o Sugar: 8g

CHAPTER 4: FRUITS AND SALADS

4.1 Thrice-bean balsamic salad

- Preparation time: 25 minutes
- Cooking time: 0 minutes
- Serving: 12

Ingredients

- 2 pounds green beans, cut into (2-inch) pieces
- 1/4 cup of sugar
- 3/4 teaspoon of salt
- 1 clove garlic, minced
- 1/2 cup of balsamic vinaigrette
- 2 cans of cannellini beans, washed and drained
- 2 cans kidney beans, washed and drained
- 4 leaves of basil, torn

Directions:

- Bring three-fourths of a Dutch oven's capacity of water to a boil. Add the green beans and simmer them till crisp-tender for 3-6 minutes, covered. Drop into icy water after draining. Drain and pat yourself dry.
- Mix the vinaigrette, salt, sugar, and garlic in a large bowl until the sugar is dissolved. Add green beans and canned beans, then toss to combine. For at least 4 hours, refrigerate covered. Immediately before serving, add basil.

Nutritional facts:

- Calories 190
- Fat: 3g
- Carbs: 33g
- Protein: 9g
- Sugar: 8g

4.2 Avocado-onion salad

- Preparation time: 15 minutes
- Cooking time: 0 minutes
- Serving: 12

Ingredients

- 1/3 cup of olive oil
- 3 medium avocados, thinly sliced
- 1/4 cup mustard, stone-ground
- 1 large (sweet) onion, thinly sliced
- 1 tablespoon of honey
- 2 tablespoons of lemon juice

Directions:

- Slices of onion and avocado should be arranged on a big dish. Mix the other ingredients in a small basin, then pour over the salad. Serve right away.

Nutritional facts:

- Calories 147
- Fat: 13g
- Carbs: 8g
- Protein: 1g
- Sugar: 3g

4.3 Chicken choppy salad

- Preparation time: 5 minutes
- Cooking time: 30 minutes
- Serving: 6

Ingredients

For the baked chicken:

- 2 pounds chicken thighs, skinless and boneless
- ½ teaspoon of pepper
- ½ teaspoon powdered onion
- ½ teaspoon powdered garlic
- ½ teaspoon of salt
- Olive oil spray

For salad:

- 3 cups kale, cut into bite-sized pieces
- 1 cup of purple cabbage, sliced
- 1 cup Brussels sprouts, cut into bite-sized slices
- 1 red onion, thinly sliced
- 1 carrot, thinly sliced
- ¼ cup of pomegranate seeds
- 1 tomato, diced
- 1 cucumber, chopped into (bite-sized) pieces
- 1 small fennel stalk, thinly sliced (divided)
- ¼ cup feta, crumbled (optional)

For garlic-citrus vinaigrette:

- ¼ cup olive oil, extra virgin
- ½ teaspoon of salt
- 1 ½ lemons, juiced
- 1 clove garlic, minced
- ½ teaspoon of pepper
- 1 teaspoon fennel, minced

Directions:

- The oven should be heated to 375°F (190°C). Season the chicken thighs on both sides, then place them in a small pan sprayed with olive oil.
- Put the pan in the oven and bake for thirty min, or until 165 degrees are registered in the thickest portion of the thigh. Place aside and let cool.
- Prepare the ingredients for the salad while the chicken bakes. Chop the kale, cucumber, and Brussels sprouts. Red onion, carrot, purple cabbage, and fennel should all be thinly sliced. Cut up the tomato. Mix the ingredients in a big bowl, then store in the fridge until required.
- In a mason jar, combine all the vinaigrette ingredients and give it a good shake. Put in the fridge until required.
- Chop the chicken into bite-sized pieces after it has cooled, then serve it over salad. Add vinaigrette and toss.

Nutritional facts:

- Calories 239
- Fat: 16g
- Carbs: 14g
- Protein: 30g
- Sugar: 5g

4.4 Watermelon-cucumber salad with mint

- Preparation time: 20 minutes
- Cooking time: 0 minutes
- Serving: 16

Ingredients

- 2 English cucumbers, sliced
- 8 cups watermelon, cubed

- 6 green-onions, chopped
- 1/4 cup of balsamic vinegar
- 1/2 teaspoon of salt
- 1/4 cup of olive oil
- 1/4 cup fresh mint, minced
- 1/2 teaspoon of pepper

Directions:

- Watermelon, cucumbers, green onions, and mint should all be combined in a big bowl. Whisk the remaining ingredients in a small dish. After adding the dressing, toss the salad. Serve right away or wait up to two hours to serve by covering it in the refrigerator.

Nutritional facts:

- Calories 60
- Fat: 3g
- Carbs: 9g
- Protein: 1g
- Sugar: 8g

4.5 Asparagus spear lemony salad

- Preparation time: 6 minutes
- Cooking time: 1 minute
- Serving: 4

Ingredients

- 1-pound asparagus spears, trimmed
- 1/4 teaspoon of salt
- 2 teaspoons of lemon juice
- 1 tablespoon of basil-pesto sauce

Directions:

- In a large skillet, cover the asparagus with water and bring it to a boil. Once boiling, cover securely and simmer for one minute or until tender-crisp.

- Asparagus should be immediately drained in a strainer and cooled with cold water. After drying the asparagus with paper towels, arrange it on a serving plate.

- The asparagus spears should be thoroughly coated with pesto before being rolled back and forth. Salt is added after the lemon juice has been drizzled. If you serve it within 30 minutes, the flavors will be at their peak.

Nutritional facts:

- Calories 40
- Fat: 2g
- Carbs: 8g
- Protein: 3g
- Sugar: 1g

4.6 Tomato artichoke toss

- Preparation time: 4 minutes
- Cooking time: 0 minutes
- Serving: 4

Ingredients

- 1 cup grape-tomatoes, halved
- 1/2 can (14-ounce) artichoke hearts, quartered and drained
- 2 ounces reduced-fat, crumbled basil feta cheese and sun-dried tomato
- 2 tablespoons Italian dressing / fat-free Caesar
- 2 tablespoons parsley, chopped (optional)

Directions:

- o Gently but thoroughly combine the tomatoes, artichoke hearts, and dressing in a medium bowl. Gently toss once more after adding the feta.
- o Serve right away or store in the fridge for up to three days, covered in plastic wrap.

Nutritional facts:

- o Calories 54
- o Fat: 2g
- o Carbs: 5g
- o Protein: 4g
- o Sugar: 2g

4.7 Creamy cucumber dill salad

- o Preparation time: 6 minutes
- o Cooking time: 0 minutes
- o Serving: 4

Ingredients

- o 1/4 cup yogurt, fat-free
- o 1/2 teaspoon dill, dried
- o 1 tablespoon mayonnaise, reduced-fat
- o 2 cups cucumber, diced
- o 1/4 teaspoon of salt

Directions:

- o In a small bowl, combine the yogurt, dill, mayonnaise, and salt and stir to combine.
- o In a mixing bowl, add the yogurt mixture and the cucumbers; gently toss to coat.
- o For the best flavors and texture, serve right away.

Nutritional facts:

- o Calories 30
- o Fat: 1g
- o Carbs: 3g
- o Protein: 1g
- o Sugar: 2g

4.8 Bean salsa salad

- o Preparation time: 6 minutes
- o Cooking time: 0 minutes
- o Serving: 4

Ingredients

- o 1 can (15-ounce) black beans, washed and drained
- o 2 tablespoons of balsamic vinegar
- o 1/4 cup red onion, finely chopped
- o 1/2 cup red-bell pepper, chopped

Directions:

- o Put everything in the bowl and toss.
- o Allow developing flavors for 15 minutes.

Nutritional facts:

- o Calories 93
- o Fat: 0g
- o Carbs: 18g
- o Protein: 6g
- o Sugar: 3g

4.9 Tangy pepper-sweet carrot salad

- o Preparation time: 12 minutes
- o Cooking time: 1 minute
- o Serving: 4

Ingredients

- o 1 1/2 cups carrots, peeled and sliced
- o 1/3 cup onion, thinly sliced
- o 3/4 cup green bell pepper, thinly sliced
- o 1/4 cup Catalina dressing, reduced-fat
- o 2 tablespoons of water

Directions:

- o In a small, microwave-safe dish, like a glass pie plate, combine the water and carrots. When the carrots are just tender-crisp, microwave them for one minute on high while covered with plastic wrap. Make sure not to overcook them; the carrots should still be somewhat crunchy.
- o The carrots should be put in a colander right away and run under cold water for about thirty seconds to cool. After shaking to drain, lay the carrots out on kitchen towels to continue to dry. Dishwasher dry.
- o Return the carrots to the dish once they have cooled fully, add the other ingredients, and gently stir to combine.
- o For a more mellowed flavor, refrigerate for 30 minutes before serving.

Nutritional facts:

- o Calories 60
- o Fat: 1g
- o Carbs: 13g
- o Protein: 1g
- o Sugar: 8g

4.10 Crispy, crunchy coleslaw

- o Preparation time: 7 minutes
- o Cooking time: 0 minutes
- o Serving: 4

Ingredients

- o 1 medium-sized green bell pepper, thinly chopped
- o 3 cups cabbage (shredded) mixed with red cabbage and carrots
- o 2 tablespoons of sugar
- o 2–3 tablespoons of apple cider vinegar
- o 1/8 teaspoon of salt

Directions:

- o All components should be combined properly by shaking them all together in a large plastic bag with a zipper.
- o Before serving, chill food for 3 hours to let flavors meld. The day you make this salad is best for serving it.

Nutritional facts:

- o Calories 46
- o Fat: 0g
- o Carbs: 11g
- o Protein: 9g
- o Sugar: 1g

4.11 Mustard-romaine salad

- o Preparation time: 5 minutes
- o Cooking time: 0 minutes
- o Serving: 4

Ingredients

- 2 teaspoons mayonnaise, reduced-fat
- 1/2 cup sour cream, fat-free
- 2 teaspoons mustard, prepared
- 1/2 teaspoon of salt
- 2 tablespoons of water
- black pepper coarsely ground to taste (optional)
- 8 cups Romaine lettuce, packed torn

Directions:

- In a small bowl, mix the water, sour cream, mayonnaise, mustard, and salt until thoroughly combined.
- Toss the lettuce with the dressing in a sizable basin until evenly coated. If desired, season with black pepper.

Nutritional facts:

- Calories 43
- Fat: 1g
- Carbs: 3g
- Protein: g
- Sugar: 3g

4.12 1,000 island wedges

- Preparation time: 5 minutes
- Cooking time: 0 minutes
- Serving: 4

Ingredients

- 1 tablespoon mayonnaise, reduced-fat
- 3 tablespoons of ketchup
- 1/2 small-head iceberg lettuce, cut into four wedges
- 1/3 cup of buttermilk, fat-free
- black pepper, coarsely ground (optional)
- 1/4 teaspoon of salt (optional)

Directions:

- In a small bowl, combine the salt, mayonnaise, and ketchup and whisk until combined. Blend completely after adding the buttermilk.
- A wedge of lettuce should be placed on each salad plate. Two tablespoons of dressing should be added to each wedge, and if preferred, black pepper should be distributed evenly.

Nutritional facts:

- Calories 42
- Fat: 2g
- Carbs: 6g
- Protein: 3g
- Sugar: 2g

4.13 Cumin and Picante salad

- Preparation time: 3 minutes
- Cooking time: 0 minutes
- Serving: 4

Ingredients

- 2 tablespoons of water
- 3/4 cup medium or mild picante sauce
- 8 cups lettuce, shredded
- 1/4 teaspoon cumin, ground
- 20 baked (bite-sized) tortilla chips, roughly crumbled

Directions:

- In a small bowl, combine the picante sauce, cumin, and water.

- Place 3 tablespoons of the picante mixture, 3 cups of lettuce, and a handful of chips on each of the 4 salad plates.

Nutritional facts:

- Calories 53
- Fat: 0g
- Carbs: 11g
- Protein: 2g
- Sugar: 1g

CHAPTER 5: SOUPS AND STEWS

5.1 Cauliflower soup

- o Preparation time: 5 minutes
- o Cooking time: 20 minutes
- o Serving: 1

Ingredients

- o 2/3 to 3/4 cup chicken broth, low-sodium, divided
- o A dash of black pepper
- o A dash of garlic powder
- o 2 bacon (lower-sodium, less-fat) slices, cooked and crumbled
- o 1-ounce cream cheese, reduced-fat
- o ⅓ cup Greek yogurt, nonfat
- o ¼ teaspoon of lemon zest
- o 1 teaspoon fresh parsley, snipped
- o 2 cups cauliflower florets, cooked

Directions:

- o Combine cauliflower, garlic powder, 2/3 cup broth, and pepper in a blender. Blend under cover until smooth.
- o Place in a compact saucepan. Just bring to a boil over medium heat. Mix in the cream cheese and as much of the rest of the broth as you need to get the consistency you want. Heat through.
- o Add yogurt, bacon, parsley, and lemon zest to the soup before serving.

Nutritional facts:

- o Calories 229

- o Fat: 10g
- o Carbs: 15g
- o Protein: 20g
- o Sugar: 9g

5.2 White bean and chicken soup

- o Preparation time: 5 minutes
- o Cooking time: 10 minutes
- o Serving: 4

Ingredients

- o 1 roasted (2-pound) chicken, shredded
- o 2 teaspoons olive oil, extra-virgin
- o 2 leeks, light green and white parts only, cut into (1/4-inch) rounds
- o 2 cans (14-ounce) chicken broth, reduced-sodium
- o 1 tablespoon sage, chopped
- o 2 cups of water
- o 1 can (15-ounce) cannellini beans, rinsed

Directions:

- o In a Dutch oven, heat the oil over medium-high heat. Leeks should be added and cooked for about 3 minutes while frequently stirring. Sage is added and cooked for another 30 seconds or until fragrant. Turn up the heat to high, stir in the broth and water, cover, and bring it to a boil. Add the beans and chicken, then simmer them for about 3 minutes, stirring regularly, with the lid on. Serve warm.

Nutritional facts:

- o Calories 248

- o Fat: 6g
- o Carbs: 14g
- o Protein: 35g
- o Sugar: 1g

5.3 Mushroom soup with sherry

- o Preparation time: 5 minutes
- o Cooking time: 5 hours 20 minutes
- o Serving: 12

Ingredients

- o 4 cups of boiling water
- o 1 tablespoon of cornstarch
- o 1 tablespoon soy sauce, lower-sodium
- o 2 cups porcini mushrooms, dried
- o 1 cup sherry, dry
- o 2 cups shallots, sliced
- o ½ teaspoon of black pepper
- o ⅝ teaspoon of kosher salt
- o 2 tablespoons of olive oil
- o 1 clove garlic, minced
- o 1 ½ tablespoons fresh thyme, chopped
- o 3 pounds assorted-fresh mushrooms, sliced
- o ⅓ cup of heavy cream

Directions:

- o The porcini mushrooms should be covered with 2 cups of boiling water. Lie still for 20 minutes. The porcini mushrooms should be drained in a colander laid over a basin while saving the mushroom broth. Pour the mushroom broth into a basin after straining it through a sieve lined with cheesecloth; discard the particles. Add the remaining 2 cups of boiling water, corn flour, soy sauce, salt, and pepper to the mushroom soup and mix well.

- o In a medium nonstick skillet, heat the oil over medium-high heat. Add the garlic and shallots; simmer, occasionally stirring, for 4 to 5 minutes or until the shallots are tender. Sherry should be added after boiling for 30 seconds. Get rid of the heat.

- o In a slow cooker, combine the fresh mushrooms, shallot combination, broth mixture, porcini mushrooms, and thyme. The vegetables should be quite soft, and the flavors should meld after 4 hours of cooking covered on HIGH. After about 20 minutes, remove the top and continue to cook until it is slightly thickened. Add a blender to two cups of the soup. Put the blender lid back on after removing the middle piece of the lid (to let steam out). Cover the aperture in the blender lid with a clean towel (to avoid splatters). Blend for 10 seconds or until smooth. Add the cream gradually after adding the puréed soup back to the slow cooker. Pour the soup into dishes and serve immediately.

Nutritional facts:

- o Calories 101
- o Fat: 5g
- o Carbs: 11g
- o Protein: 5g
- o Sugar: 4g

5.4 Wild rice and turkey soup

- o Preparation time: 5 minutes
- o Cooking time: 30 minutes
- o Serving: 4

Ingredients

- o 1 tablespoon olive oil, extra-virgin
- o 2 cups mushrooms, sliced
- o ¼ cup shallots, chopped
- o ¾ cup carrots, chopped
- o ¾ cup celery, chopped
- o ¼ cup of all-purpose flour
- o 4 cups chicken broth, reduced-sodium
- o ½ cup sour cream, reduced-fat
- o ¼ teaspoon pepper, freshly ground
- o 3 cups chicken/ turkey, cooked and shredded
- o 2 tablespoons parsley, chopped fresh
- o 1 cup rice, quick-cooking
- o ¼ teaspoon of salt

Directions:

- o Oil is heated in a big pot over medium heat. Add the mushrooms, celery, carrots, and shallots; stir-fry for about 5 minutes or until the vegetables are tender. Cook for a further 2 minutes while whisking in the flour, salt, and pepper.

- o While scraping off any browned bits, add the stock and bring it to a boil. Reduce the heat to a low simmer and add the rice. For 5 to 7 minutes, cook the rice with the cover on. Stir in the chicken (or turkey), sour cream, and

parsley; cook for an additional 2 minutes or until well cooked.

Nutritional facts:

- o Calories 378
- o Fat: 10g
- o Carbs: 28g
- o Protein: 36g
- o Sugar: 2.8g

5.5 Tomato and pepper soup

- o Preparation time: 5 minutes
- o Cooking time: 32 minutes
- o Serving: 4

Ingredients

- o 14 .5-ounce can think of tomatoes, stewed
- o 15 .5-ounce can think of navy beans, rinsed and drained
- o 1/2–1 medium chipotle-chili-pepper in adobo sauce, finely chopped
- o 8 ounces onion and pepper stir-fry
- o 1 cup of water
- o 1/4 teaspoon of salt

Directions:

- o The tomatoes, chipotle pepper, peppers, and water should be combined in a big pot. Using high heat, bring to a boil.

- o Onions should be soft after 25 minutes of simmering, so lower the heat, cover securely, and stir occasionally.

- o With a fork, mash the larger tomato pieces. Add the salt and beans, and cook for an additional 5 minutes.

Nutritional facts:

- Calories 151
- Fat: 1g
- Carbs: 30g
- Protein: 8g
- Sugar: 6g

5.6 Very soup

- Preparation time: 2 minutes
- Cooking time: 15 minutes
- Serving: 4

Ingredients

- 4 ounces (50% reduced-fat) pork sausage
- 14 .5-ounce can of tomatoes stewed in liquid
- 2 cups green cabbage, coarsely chopped
- 10-ounce package of mixed vegetables, frozen
- 1 1/2 cups of water

Directions:

- Heat up a sizable pot over medium-high heat. Spray nonstick cooking spray on the pan, then add the sausage. While cooking, break up large pieces of sausage and often toss until it is no longer pink. Place aside on a different platter.
- Apply nonstick cooking spray once more to the pan, add the cabbage, and simmer for 3 minutes while tossing constantly. Bring to a boil the remaining ingredients after adding them. When the vegetables are

cooked, turn down the heat, cover securely, and simmer for 10 minutes.

- Take the dish off the heat, add the sausage, cover it, and let it stand for five minutes so the flavors may meld.

Nutritional facts:

- Calories 143
- Fat: 6g
- Carbs: 18g
- Protein: 8g
- Sugar: 7g

5.7 Green pepper soup

- Preparation time: 5 minutes
- Cooking time: 25 minutes
- Serving: 4

Ingredients

- 1 pound (90% lean) beef, ground
- 1 packet (0.25-ounce) of chili-seasoning mix
- 1 large green bell pepper, chopped
- 14 .5-ounce can of tomatoes stewed in liquid
- 3/4 cup of water

Directions:

- A big nonstick skillet should be heated up over medium-high heat. Apply nonstick cooking spray to the skillet, add the meat, and heat, constantly tossing, until the steak is no longer pink. Placed aside on a different platter.
- Coat the pan again with non-stick cooking spray. Add the peppers, and

- cook, often stirring, for 5 min or until the edges start to brown

- Bring the skillet's contents to a boil after adding the last few ingredients. Reduce the heat, tightly cover the pot, and simmer for 15 minutes or until the peppers are very soft. Stirring occasionally, crush the tomatoes with the back of a spoon as they cook.

- Remove from heat and set aside for 10 minutes to allow flavors to develop.

Nutritional facts:

- Calories 244
- Fat: 10g
- Carbs: 14g
- Protein: 24g
- Sugar: 4g

5.8 Sweet corn and peppers soup

- Preparation time: 5 minutes
- Cooking time: 20 minutes
- Serving: 55

Ingredients

- 1 pound onion and pepper, stir-fry
- 10 ounces corn kernels, frozen and thawed
- 2 ounces processed (reduced-fat) cheese, cubes
- 1 1/4 cups milk, fat-free
- 1/8 teaspoon of black pepper
- 1/2 teaspoon of salt
- 1 cup of water

Directions:

- Put the water on high heat in a big pot to get it to a boil. Regain a boil after adding the peppers When the onions are ready, turn down the heat, cover securely, and simmer for 15 minutes.

- Add the milk and corn. Bring to a boil over high heat, then immediately turn off the heat.

- Let the cheese melt and the flavors meld by adding the remaining ingredients, covering, and setting aside for 5 minutes.

Nutritional facts:

- Calories 117
- Fat: 2g
- Carbs: 21g
- Protein: 7g
- Sugar: 8g

5.9 Green onion and cream potato soup

- Preparation time: 10 minutes
- Cooking time: 15 minutes
- Serving: 3

Ingredients

- 2 cups milk, fat-free
- 3 tablespoons margarine, reduced-fat
- 1 pound of baking potatoes, diced
- 1/4 teaspoon of black pepper
- 1/2 teaspoon of salt
- 3 tablespoons green (green and white parts) onions, finely chopped

Directions:

- In a big pot over high heat, just bring the milk to just a boil.

- o Just bring to a boil again after adding the potatoes. Reduce the heat to low, cover, and cook for 12 minutes or till the potatoes are soft.
- o Add the margarine, pepper, and salt after taking the pan off the heat. Mash the mixture with a whisk, a potato masher, or a hand-held electric mixer until thickened but still lumpy.

Nutritional facts:

- o Calories 204
- o Fat: 5g
- o Carbs: 32g
- o Protein: 8g
- o Sugar: 10g

5.10 Green peppers tilapia stew

- o Preparation time: 10 minutes
- o Cooking time: 40 minutes
- o Serving: 4

Ingredients

- o 1 medium green bell pepper, chopped
- o 1 pound of tilapia filets, 1-inch pieces
- o 14 .5-ounce can consist of tomatoes stewed with Italian-seasonings
- o 1/8 teaspoon of salt
- o 3/4 teaspoon of seafood seasoning
- o 1 cup of water

Directions:

- o Heat up a sizable pot over medium heat. Spray the pan with non-stick cooking spray. Add the bell pepper and cook for 5 minutes, tossing periodically or until the bell pepper starts to brown softly.
- o Increase the heat to high, add the tomatoes, and then boil. Reduce heat, cover, and simmer for 25 minutes or until tomatoes are soft. Tear apart the tomatoes with the spoon's back.
- o Stir carefully after adding the fish and seasonings. Just bring it to a boil after turning up the heat to high. Turn down the heat, cover closely, and simmer the fish for three minutes or until the center is opaque. Remove from the fire and leave covered for 10 minutes to let the flavors meld.

Nutritional facts:

- o Calories 147
- o Fat: 3g
- o Carbs: 8g
- o Protein: 24g
- o Sugar: 5g

5.11 Minestrone soup

- o Preparation time: 10 minutes
- o Cooking time: 6-8 hours 30 minutes
- o Serving: 8

Ingredients

- o 4 carrots, chopped
- o 3 garlic cloves, minced
- o 3 stalks of celery, chopped
- o 1 (small) red onion, chopped
- o 2 cups green beans, cut into (2-inch) pieces
- o 2 cans (15 ounces) tomatoes, diced

- o 2 cans (15 ounces) of red kidney beans without sodium
- o 6 cups vegetable broth without sodium
- o 1 teaspoon red pepper, crushed
- o 2 tablespoons of Italian seasoning
- o ½ teaspoon pepper, ground
- o ¾ teaspoon of salt, divided
- o 4 ounces (whole-wheat) pasta elbows
- o 1 (large) zucchini, chopped
- o ½ cup Parmesan cheese, freshly grated

Directions:

- o In a 6- to 8-qt slow cooker, combine the following ingredients: celery, carrots, onion, green beans, garlic, tomatoes, broth, crushed red pepper, kidney beans, Italian seasoning, 1/4 teaspoon salt, and pepper. Cook for 6-8 hours on Low, covered.
- o Add the remaining half teaspoon of salt along with the pasta and zucchini. For a further 15 to 20 minutes, simmer the pasta on Low with the cover on. Serve immediately, adding roughly 1 1/2 tbsp. to each serving. Parmesan.

Nutritional facts:

- o Calories 222
- o Fat: 2g
- o Carbs: 41g
- o Protein: 11g
- o Sugar: 10g

5.12 Potato soup

- o Preparation time: 10 minutes
- o Cooking time: 20 minutes
- o Serving: 5

Ingredients

- o 2 bacon slices, halved
- o 1 tablespoon of butter
- o 1 ½ pounds potatoes, diced
- o 2 cups chicken broth, low-sodium
- o ½ cup onion, chopped
- o ½ cup of sour cream
- o ½ cup cheddar cheese, shredded and divided
- o ¼ teaspoon of pepper
- o ½ teaspoon of salt
- o ¼ cup chives or scallion greens

Directions:

- o In a multicooker, add the butter, and heat on the sauté setting until melted. Cook the bacon for 4 to 5 minutes, stirring periodically, until crisp. Bacon and butter drippings are left in the pot after being transferred to a clean towel to drain. Add the onion to the multicooker, and cook it for two to three minutes while stirring. Add broth and potatoes. Cut the heat off. Lock the lid by closing it. Cook for 10 minutes under high pressure.
- o Let go of the tension. With an immersion blender, puree the soup until nearly smooth but slightly lumpy. (Alternatively, you might use a food processor to purée the soup. When combining hot liquids, exercise

caution.) Stir in the sour cream until it is smooth. Add salt, pepper, and 1/4 cup of cheese. Stir the cheese until it has melted. Serve with the leftover 1/4 cup cheese, bacon bits, and scallion greens as garnishes (or chives).

Nutritional facts:

- Calories 87
- Fat: 4g
- Carbs: 10g
- Protein: 3g
- Sugar: 0.9g

5.13 Rutabaga stew

- Preparation time: 20 minutes
- Cooking time: 4 hours 5 minutes
- Serving: 15

Ingredients

- 1 ½ pounds chicken, diced
- 1 tablespoon of vegetable oil
- 4 rutabagas, diced
- 4 carrots, diced
- 4 medium-sized beets, diced
- 1 (red) onion, diced
- 3 celery stalks, diced
- water, as required

Directions:

- In a Dutch oven or sizable pot, heat the vegetable oil over medium-low heat. In heated oil, cook chicken for 3 to 5 minutes, frequently stirring, until thoroughly browned.
- To the pot, add beets, rutabagas, carrots, celery, and onion.

- Give the vegetable mixture a thorough covering of water. Reduce the heat to low and keep the vegetables submerged in water for a minimum of 4 hours.

Nutritional facts:

- Calories 111
- Fat: 2g
- Carbs: 13g
- Protein: 11g
- Sugar: 9g

5.14 Mango Gazpacho

- Preparation time: 10 minutes
- Cooking time: 0 minutes
- Serving: 6

Ingredients

- 2 tablespoons olive oil, extra-virgin
- 2 cups fresh mangoes, sliced into 1/4-inch diced
- 1 onion, cut into (1/4-inch) dice
- 2 cups of orange juice
- 1 cucumber, sliced into (1/4-inch) dice
- 1 red bell pepper, cut into (1/4-inch) dice
- 2 tablespoons fresh basil, cilantro or parsley, chopped
- 2 medium-sized cloves of garlic, minced
- 3 tablespoons of lime juice
- 1 jalapeno pepper, minced (Optional)
- Salt and black pepper, to taste

Directions:

- Mangoes, orange juice, and oil should be blended in a food processor or blender. Add to a mixing bowl with the rest of the ingredients. To taste, add pepper and salt to the food. Keep chilled until you're ready to serve. (Can be prepared up to a day ahead of serving).

Nutritional facts:

- o   Calories 147
- o   Fat: 5g
- o   Carbs: 26g
- o   Protein: 2g
- o   Sugar: 20g

CHAPTER 6: MEAT RECIPES

6.1 Beef tenderloin

- o   Preparation time: 3 minutes
- o   Cooking time: 11 minutes
- o   Serving: 4

Ingredients

- o   4 beef (5-ounce) tenderloin steaks, about (3/4-inch) thick, fat removed
- o   1/4 teaspoon black pepper, coarsely ground
- o   1/2 teaspoon of beef bouillon, granules
- o   2 teaspoons of Worcestershire sauce
- o   1 garlic clove, large split
- o   1/2 cup of water
- o   1/4 teaspoon of salt

Directions:

- o   Rub the garlic clove on the beef. A big nonstick skillet should be heated up over medium- high heat. Cook the meat in the skillet for three minutes

after spraying it with nonstick cooking spray. Cook for 2 more minutes after turning.

- o   Turning once, cook the steaks for an additional 4 minutes at medium-low heat or till they are cooked to your liking. Placed aside on a different platter.

- o   The mixture should boil for 1 minute or until it contains 1/4 cup of liquid after increasing the heat to medium-high, adding the additional ingredients, and bringing it to a boil. Over the beef, pour the juices.

Nutritional facts:

- o   Calories 180
- o   Fat: 7g
- o   Carbs: 1g
- o   Protein: 26g
- o   Sugar: 1g

6.2 Southwest-style grilled steak with vibrant skillet veggies

- o   Preparation time: 10 minutes
- o   Cooking time: 30 minutes
- o   Serving: 1-2

Ingredients

- o   1 beef Steak, cut (1 inch) thick

Marinade

- o   1 tablespoon garlic, chopped
- o   1/4 cup lime juice
- o   1 teaspoon cumin, ground
- o   1 tablespoon of olive oil
- o   1/2 teaspoon black pepper, coarse grind

- o 1/4 cup mild salsa, prepared

Colorful Vegetables

- o 1 medium (red or green) bell pepper, cut into (1/4 inch) strips

- o 2 cups zucchini, sliced into (1/4-inch) thick

- o 8 ounces button mushrooms, sliced (1/4- inch) thick

- o 3/4 teaspoon cumin, ground

- o 1/2 teaspoon of salt

- o 1/4 teaspoon black pepper, coarse grind

- o 1/4 cup green onions, chopped

- o 1 cup tomatoes, finely chopped

- o 2 tablespoons of olive oil

Directions:

- o In a small bowl, combine the marinade ingredients. In a food-safe plastic bag, combine the marinade and the beef steak; turn to coat.

- o Marinate in the refrigerator for 6 hours or even overnight while turning the bag occasionally.

- o Take the steak out of the marinade and discard it.

- o Steak should be placed on the grid over medium, ash-coated coals. For rare, medium doneness (145F), grill covered for 13 to 15 minutes (under medium heat on a preheated gas grill, 17 to 20 minutes) and turn once. Avoid overcooking.

- o Prepare the colorful vegetables in the meanwhile. 2 tablespoons of olive oil are heated over medium-high heat in a sizable nonstick skillet.

- o Add the bell pepper strips and cook, frequently stirring, for 1 to 2 minutes or until crisp-tender.

- o When the vegetables are crisp-tender, add the mushrooms, zucchini, cumin, salt, and black pepper. Cook and stir for 3 to 4 minutes.

- o For one minute, while stirring, add the tomato and green onion.

- o Slice the meat very thinly and add salt to taste. Serve alongside vibrant vegetables.

Nutritional facts:

- o Calories 277

- o Fat: 13g

- o Carbs: 8g

- o Protein: 33g

- o Sugar: 2g

6.3 Simple meatballs

- o Preparation time: 15 minutes

- o Cooking time: 30 minutes

- o Serving: 6

Ingredients

- o 1 pound (90% lean) beef, ground

- o 3 (large) egg whites

- o 1/2 cup oats, quick-cooking

- o 26 .5-ounce jar (meatless) spaghetti sauce, divided

- o 1 tablespoon basil, dried (optional)

Directions:

- o In a sizable bowl, combine the oats, basil, ground beef, egg whites, and ½ cup of spaghetti sauce. 24 1-inch meatballs should be formed from the ingredients.

- o A big nonstick skillet should be heated up over medium-high heat. Spray the pan with nonstick cooking spray. Add the meatballs, and cook, constantly tossing, until browned. When stir-frying, use 2 utensils to stir.

- o Adding the remaining spaghetti sauce, heat just until it begins to boil. Simmer for 20 minutes on a lower heat with a tight lid.

Nutritional facts:

- o Calories 278
- o Fat: 10g
- o Carbs: 13g
- o Protein: 20g
- o Sugar: 13g

6.4 Beef with sweet ginger sauce

- o Preparation time: 4 minutes
- o Cooking time: 4 minutes
- o Serving: 4

Ingredients

- o 2 tablespoons soy sauce
- o 2 teaspoons ginger root, grated
- o 1 tablespoon of sugar
- o 1 pound sirloin steak, cut into strips

Directions:

- o In a small bowl, combine the sugar, soy sauce, and gingerroot; leave aside.

- o Heat a sizable nonstick pan on medium-high. Apply nonstick cooking spray to the skillet, add half the meat, and cook for 1 minute while stirring regularly.

- o The beef should be taken out of the skillet and placed on a separate platter. Apply nonstick cooking spray once more to the skillet and fry the remaining steak for 1 minute.

- o Add the soy sauce to the skillet with the initial batch of beef.

Nutritional facts:

- o Calories 244
- o Fat: 6g
- o Carbs: 4g
- o Protein: 42g
- o Sugar: 4g

6.5 Sirloin hoagies

- o Preparation time: 12 minutes
- o Cooking time: 16 minutes
- o Serving: 4

Ingredients

- o 1 pound sirloin steak, boneless
- o 1/4 teaspoon of salt, divided
- o 1 (large) onion, thinly sliced
- o 8 ounces of bread, whole wheat
- o 1/2 cup of water
- o 1 1/2 tablespoons of prepared mustard
- o 1/2 teaspoon of black pepper

Directions:

- o Set the oven's temperature to 350.

- On each side of the steak, evenly distribute the pepper and 1/8 teaspoon of salt. A big nonstick skillet should be heated up over medium-high heat. Cook the steak in the skillet for 5 minutes after spraying with nonstick cooking spray.

- Once again, heat for 4 more minutes or until the steak is cooked to your preferences. On a chopping board, place the beef; then, set it aside.

- After lowering the heat to medium, add the onions to the nonstick cooking spray-coated pan drippings. Apply nonstick frying spray to the onions, then heat them for 6-7 minutes, stirring frequently, or until they are deeply browned.

- While stirring continuously, add water to the onions and simmer for one minute or until the majority of the excess water has evaporated. Get rid of the heat.

- Place the bread in the oven, wrap it in foil, and bake for five minutes or until heated. Meanwhile, cut the beef into thin, diagonal slices.

- The bread should be divided lengthwise using a serrated knife. Each cut side should then have a small layer of mustard applied. Beef is placed on top, followed by onions and any liquids. The remaining salt over the steak, top with the remaining bread half and then cut into fourths crosswise.

Nutritional facts:

- Calories 317

- Fat: 6g

- Carbs: 36g

- Protein: 28g

- Sugar: 6g

6.6 Beefy patties with grilled onions

- Preparation time: 7 minutes

- Cooking time: 15 minutes

- Serving: 4

Ingredients

- 1 pound (90% lean) beef, ground

- 1 large (yellow) onion, thinly sliced

- 2 tablespoons (Ranch-style)) salad dressing and seasoning-mix

- 1/4 cup of water

- 1 tablespoon of Dijon mustard

Directions:

- In a medium bowl, combine the mustard, salad dressing mix, and ground beef. 4 patties made with the beef mixture.

- A big nonstick skillet should be heated up over medium-high heat. Add the onions after spraying the skillet with non-stick cooking spray. Apply nonstick frying spray to the onions and heat for 7 minutes, stirring regularly, or till they are deeply browned. On a different platter, place them away.

- Reapply nonstick cooking spray to the skillet, add the patties, and cook for 4 minutes. The patties should no longer be pink in the center after 3 minutes of flipping them. Put them on a plate for serving.

- After adding the water and onion to the drippings in the pan, heat for thirty seconds while scraping the sides and sides of the pan, and spoon the mixture over the patties once it has slightly thickened.

Nutritional facts:

- Calories 215
- Fat: 9g
- Carbs: 8g
- Protein: 23g
- Sugar: 3g

6.7 Cumin-seasoned beef patties

- Preparation time: 5 minutes
- Cooking time: 8 minutes
- Serving: 4

Ingredients

- 1 pound (90% lean) beef, ground
- 2 teaspoons cumin, ground
- 1/8 teaspoon of black pepper
- 1/4 teaspoon salt, divided
- 1/3 cup mild-picante sauce, divided
- 1/4 cup sour cream, fat-free

Directions:

- In a medium bowl, in a medium bowl, combine cumin, ground beef, 2 tbsps. of Picante sauce, 1/8 tsp. salt, and black pepper. Make 4 patties out of the beef mixture.

- A big nonstick skillet should be heated up over medium-high heat. Apply nonstick cooking spray to the skillet, add patties, and fry for 4 minutes. The patties should no longer be pink in the center after 3 minutes of flipping them.

- In the meantime, combine the sour cream, 2 tbsp. picante sauce, and 1/8 teaspoon salt in a small bowl.

- Add 1 1/2 tablespoons of sour cream to each patty. If preferred, add an extra 1/2 teaspoon of picante sauce to each serving.

Nutritional facts:

- Calories 200
- Fat: 10g
- Carbs: 2g
- Protein: 23g
- Sugar: 1g

6.8 Chili-stuffed potatoes

- Preparation time: 5 minutes
- Cooking time: 10 minutes
- Serving: 4

Ingredients

- 12 ounces (90% lean) beef, ground
- 4 (8-ounce) baking potatoes, pierced with a fork
- 1 packet (0.25-ounce) chili-seasoning mix
- 1/2 cup sour cream, reduced-fat
- 1/4 teaspoon of salt
- cheddar cheese, reduced-fat (optional)
- 3/4 cup of water

Directions:

- The potatoes should be microwaved on high for 10 to 11 minutes or until a fork can easily pierce them.

- In the meantime, heat up a sizable nonstick skillet over medium-high heat. Apply nonstick cooking spray to the skillet, add the meat, and heat, constantly tossing, until the steak is no longer pink.

- Stir in the water and chili spice. Cook for one to two minutes or until thick.

- Half a cup of chili should be spooned onto each potato after it has been almost completely cut in half, and it should be topped with cheese or sour cream (if using).

Nutritional facts:

- Calories 333
- Fat: 8g
- Carbs: 44g
- Protein: 22g
- Sugar: 3g

6.9 Onion roast

- Preparation time: 20 minutes
- Cooking time: 1 hour 10 minutes
- Serving: 6

Ingredients

- 1 3/4 pound lean roast, round
- 2 medium onions, sliced in (1/2-inch) wedges and divided
- 1 pound carrots, quartered lengthwise and sliced into (3-inch) pieces
- 1-ounce packet of onion soup mix
- 1/4 cup of water

Directions:

- Set the oven's temperature to 325.

- The carrots and onions should be arranged on a 13 x 9-inch nonstick baking sheet that has been coated with nonstick cooking spray.

- Bring a medium skillet to a boil over medium-high heat. Apply nonstick cooking spray to the skillet, add the meat, and brown for 2 minutes. 2 minutes later, turn and continue to brown.

- Over the vegetables in the middle of the baking pan, put the beef. Pouring the water over the steak after scraping up the pan drippings. Sprinkle the soup mix evenly.

- Cook for 1 hour and 5 minutes, or until a beef thermometer reads 135 degrees, with the pan tightly covered with foil. Before slicing the meat, let it rest for 15 minutes on a chopping board. While the beef is standing, the temperature will increase by another 10 degrees.

- To keep the vegetables warm, keep the pan covered. Place the beef pieces, vegetables, and pan liquids all on a serving tray. Distribute the pan liquids over the steak.

Nutritional facts:

- Calories 229
- Fat: 5g
- Carbs: 13g
- Protein: 32g
- Sugar: 7g

6.10 Bourbon-filet mignon

- Preparation time: 5 minutes

- o Cooking time: 12 minutes
- o Serving: 4

Ingredients

- o 4 filets (5-ounce) mignon steaks, about (¾ inch) thick, fat removed
- o 1/8–1/4 teaspoon black pepper, coarsely ground
- o 1/2 teaspoon of salt divided
- o 1/2 cup coffee
- o 2 teaspoons of Worcestershire sauce
- o 2 tablespoons of bourbon

Directions:

- o Allow the meat to rest for 15 minutes after sprinkling it with 1/4 tsp salt and pepper on both sides.
- o Set the oven temperature to 200 degrees.
- o In the meantime, combine in a small bowl the bourbon, coffee, Worcestershire sauce, and 1/4 tsp salt.
- o Until it is heated, place a sizable non-stick skillet over high heat.
- o Apply nonstick cooking spray to the skillet. Add the steaks, and heat for 3 min on each side.
- o To cook the steaks to the desired doneness, lower the heat to medium-low and cook them for an additional 2 to 6 minutes. Place them in the oven on separate dinner plates.
- o The coffee mixture should be added to the skillet and cooked for 2 minutes on high heat or until it is reduced to 2 tbsp. Serve the beef right away after spooning the sauce over it evenly.

Nutritional facts.

- o Calories 195
- o Fat: 7g
- o Carbs: 1g
- o Protein: 26g
- o Sugar: 1g

6.11 Beef stewed and ale

- o Preparation time: 5 minutes
- o Cooking time: 1 hour 40 minutes
- o Serving: 4

Ingredients

- o 1 pound top-round steak, cut in (1/4 inch×3 1/2 inch)strips
- o 14 .5-ounce can consist of tomatoes stewed
- o 1 cup onion, chopped
- o 1 cup of beer
- o 1/4 teaspoon of black pepper
- o 1/4 teaspoon of salt
- o 1 teaspoon of sugar (optional)

Directions:

- o A big nonstick skillet should be heated up over medium-high heat. Spray some nonstick cooking spray on the skillet. Put half the beef strips in 2 batches, brown them while turning constantly, and then set them aside on a different platter. The other beef strips are in the same manner.
- o Onions should be added to a nonstick skillet that has been freshly coated with cooking spray. Cook for 4

minutes, stirring periodically, till the onions are transparent. Add the steak and any accumulated juices, along with the remaining ingredients.

- o Over high heat, bring to a boil. Then, lower the heat, cover securely, and simmer for one hour and thirty minutes or till the beef is extremely soft. Mash the beef bits with the bottom of a spoon to slightly thicken the dish.

Nutritional facts:

- o Calories 183
- o Fat: 3g
- o Carbs: 13g
- o Protein: 25g
- o Sugar: 6g

6.12 Steak fajitas (Air-fryer)

- o Preparation time: 15 minutes
- o Cooking time: 15 minutes
- o Serving: 6

Ingredients

- o 1/2 cup red onion, diced
- o 2 (large) tomatoes, chopped
- o 1/4 cup of lime juice
- o 3 tablespoons cilantro, minced fresh
- o 1 jalapeno pepper, minced
- o 3/4 teaspoon of salt, divided
- o 2 teaspoons cumin, ground and divided
- o 1 flank beef steak
- o 1 (large) onion, sliced

- o lime wedges and sliced avocado (Optional)
- o 6 tortillas (8 inches), whole wheat

Directions:

- o Put the first five ingredients for the salsa in a small dish and add 1 tsp. salt and 1/4 tsp. cumin. Let stand till serving.

- o The air fryer should be heated to 400 °F. Add salt and leftover cumin to the steak. In the air-fryer basket, place it on a greased surface. Cook for 6 to 8 minutes on each side or until the meat is the required doneness (for moderate, a thermometer must read 135°; for medium, 140°; and for medium-well, 145°). Take it out of the basket, then stand for five minutes.

- o Meanwhile, put an onion in the air fryer basket on a tray. Cook for 2-3 minutes, stirring once, until crisp-tender. Serve steak in tortillas with salsa and onion after thinly slicing it against the grain. Serve with wedges of lime and avocado, if desired.

Nutritional facts:

- o Calories 309
- o Fat: 9g
- o Carbs: 29g
- o Protein: 27g
- o Sugar: 3g

6.13 Tendered green pepper

- o Preparation time: 10 minutes
- o Cooking time: 60 minutes
- o Serving: 4

Ingredients

- 1 pound top-round steak, cut into (4 equal) pieces
- 1/4 cup of ketchup
- 1 cup of water
- 2 medium (green) bell peppers, thin strips
- 1/4 teaspoon of black pepper
- 1/2 teaspoon of salt
- 1/4 cup Italian salad dressing, fat-free

Directions:

- In a sizable zipped plastic bag, combine the steak and salad dressing. Seal firmly and shake vigorously to distribute the coating evenly. Turning occasionally, chill for at least 8 hours in the refrigerator.

- In a small bowl, combine the ketchup, water, salt, and pepper; leave aside.

- A big nonstick skillet should be heated up over medium-high heat. Spray some nonstick cooking spray on the skillet. Steaks are placed in the skillet once the meat is taken out of the marinade and the marinade is discarded. Cook for 3 minutes, turn and cook for an additional 2 minutes.

- Turning once, cook the steaks for an additional 4 minutes at medium-low heat or till they are cooked to your liking. Pour the ketchup sauce over everything after adding the green peppers. Bring to a boil, lower heat, cover closely, and simmer for approximately 55 minutes or until very tender.

Nutritional facts:

- Calories 167
- Fat: 3g
- Carbs: 9g
- Protein: 24g
- Sugar: 5g

6.14 Spicy sirloin steak

- Preparation time: 2 minutes
- Cooking time: 11 minutes
- Serving: 4

Ingredients

- 1 pound sirloin steak, boneless and remove fat
- 1/8 teaspoon of salt
- 2 tablespoons of chili seasoning

Directions:

- Sprinkle the chili seasoning blend over the sirloin and rub it in on both sides. For a spicier flavor, let stand for 15 minutes or overnight in the refrigerator (Wait 15 minutes before grilling steak at room temperature).

- A big nonstick skillet should be heated up over medium-high heat. Apply nonstick cooking spray to the skillet. Add the beef, and heat for 5 minutes. Cook the steak for five minutes after turning it and lowering the heat to medium. Avoid overcooking. Take the skillet off the heat, cover it, and let it stand for 2 minutes.

- Slice the meat into 1/4-inch pieces after salting it. Any remaining liquids should be poured over the meat slices.

Nutritional facts:

- Calories 148
- Fat: 4g
- Carbs: 2g
- Protein: 24g
- Sugar: 0g

6.15 Pork chops

- Preparation time: 3 minutes
- Cooking time: 12 minutes
- Serving: 4

Ingredients

- 1 tablespoon dried (Italian) salad dressing and recipe mix
- 4 (4-ounce) pork chops, boneless and fat removed

Directions:

- Apply the salad dressing mixture evenly to the pork chops' two sides, gently pushing down to help the spices stick.
- A big nonstick skillet should be heated up over medium heat. Apply nonstick cooking spray to the skillet. Add the pork, and heat for 4 minutes. Turn the pork over and cook for a further 4 minutes or until the middle is just barely pink.
- Turn off the heat and leave the pork in the skillet for two to three minutes or until some of the juices start to come out. To remove the pan residue, repeatedly stir the pork chunks in the skillet.

Nutritional facts:

- Calories 159
- Fat: 7g

- Carbs: 1g
- Protein: 21g
- Sugar: 1g

6.16 Pork with rice

- Preparation time: 9 minutes
- Cooking time: 8 minutes
- Serving: 4

Ingredients

- 12 small olives, coarsely chopped
- 1/3 cup medium-salsa
- 4 (4-ounce) pork chops, boneless
- 1/4 teaspoon of black pepper
- 1/4 teaspoon of salt
- 1/2 cup of water
- 2 cups brown rice, cooked

Directions:

- Gently combine the cooked rice with the salsa and olives. To keep warm, put it on a serving tray and wrap it with a foil sheet.
- A big nonstick skillet should be heated up over medium-high heat. Spray some nonstick cooking spray on the skillet. Add salt and pepper to the pork. Immediately lower the heat to medium-low after adding the pork to the skillet, and cook for 4 minutes. Turn the pork over and cook for a further 4 minutes or until the middle is just barely pink. Lay the pork over the rice, wrap it in foil, and set it aside.
- Bring the water to a boil in the skillet over medium-high heat, stirring constantly. Boil for 2 minutes or until

1/4 cup of liquid remains. Put the sauce on the rice and pork.

Nutritional facts:

- o Calories 279
- o Fat: 9g
- o Carbs: 20g
- o Protein: 24g
- o Sugar: 1g

CHAPTER 7: POULTRY AND CHICKEN

7.1 Molasses drumsticks

- o Preparation time: 10 minutes
- o Cooking time: 25 minutes
- o Serving: 4

Ingredients

- o 2 tablespoons of dark molasses
- o 1/4 cup soy sauce
- o 8 chicken drumsticks, washed and patted dry
- o 2 tablespoons of lime juice

Directions:

- o In a small bowl, combine the lime juice and soy sauce and stir until well combined.
- o Put the drumsticks inside a large plastic bag with a zipper. Add 3 tbsp of soy sauce mix to the bag. Shake the container vigorously to distribute the coating over the chicken. Turning occasionally, chill for at least two hours in the refrigerator.
- o The leftover soy sauce mixture should now include molasses. Cover it with plastic wrap and store it in the fridge until required.
- o Set the broiler to high. Put the drumsticks on the rack and spray the pan and broiler rack with nonstick cooking spray. Discard the marinade that was in the bag. Drumsticks should be broiler-broiled for 25 minutes, rotating every 5 minutes or until the center is no longer pink.

- o The drumsticks should be put in a big basin. Pouring the saved soy sauce mixture over the drumsticks after stirring it. Allow the drumsticks to remain for 3 minutes to absorb seasonings after gently tossing them to coat evenly.

Nutritional facts:

- o Calories 226
- o Fat: 6g
- o Carbs: 8g
- o Protein: 32g
- o Sugar: 7g

7.2 Lemon Greek chicken

- o Preparation time: 15 minutes
- o Cooking time: 50 minutes
- o Serving: 4

Ingredients

- o 2 teaspoons olive oil, extra virgin
- o 8 chicken drumsticks, washed and patted dry
- o 1 teaspoon of lemon zest
- o 4 tablespoons of lemon juice, divided
- o 1/2 teaspoon of salt (optional)
- o 2 tablespoons Greek seasoning, dried

Directions:

- o In a gallon-sized zipped plastic bag, combine the drumsticks, lemon zest, olive oil, Greek seasoning, and 2 tbsp lemon juice. To uniformly coat the chicken, close the bag and shake it back and forth. Turning occasionally, place in refrigerator for 8 hours to 48 hours.

- o Set the oven's temperature to 350.

- o Pour the marinade equally over the drumsticks and arrange them in a single layer in a 12 x 8-inch baking dish that has been coated with nonstick cooking spray. Bake the drumsticks, turning them regularly, for 50 to 55 minutes or until the middle is no longer pink.

- o The drumsticks should be put on a serving plate. In a small bowl, combine the 2 tbsp lemon juice and salt (if using), then pour the mixture equally over the chicken pieces.

Nutritional facts:

- o Calories 179
- o Fat: 7g
- o Carbs: 2g
- o Protein: 25g
- o Sugar: 1g

7.3 Chicken lemon pasta

- o Preparation time: 5 minutes
- o Cooking time: 10 minutes
- o Serving: 1

Ingredients

- o 2 teaspoons olive oil, extra-virgin
- o 1 cup of baby spinach
- o 1 cup zucchini, spiralized
- o ½ cup rotisserie-chicken breast, shredded
- o ⅛ teaspoon pepper, ground
- o ⅛ teaspoon of salt
- o 2 tablespoons Parmesan cheese, grated

- o 1 tablespoon of lemon juice
- o 1 teaspoon lemon zest, grated
- o 1 tablespoon of panko breadcrumbs, toasted
- o ½ cup (whole-wheat) spaghetti, cooked

Directions:

- o Over medium heat, warm the oil in a sizable nonstick skillet. For one minute, add the zucchini. Cook for another minute after adding the chicken and spinach. Add salt and pepper, then turn off the heat. Add the cooked spaghetti, lemon zest and, juice, Parmesan and blend. Serve after adding toasted panko.

Nutritional facts:

- o Calories 350
- o Fat: 15g
- o Carbs: 26g
- o Protein: 28g
- o Sugar: 3g

7.4 Barbecued peachy chicken

- o Preparation time: 15 minutes
- o Cooking time: 18 minutes
- o Serving: 4

Ingredients

- o 8 chicken drumsticks, washed and patted dry
- o 2 teaspoons ginger root, grated
- o 1/2 cup of barbeque sauce
- o 1/4 cup peach (all-fruit) spread

Directions:

- o Set the broiler to high.

- Coat a rack for the broiler and a pan with cooking spray that won't stick. Place the drumsticks over the grill and broil them for 8 minutes, about 4 inches from the heat source. The juices should run clear after 6 minutes of turning and broiling.

- In the meantime, microwave the fruit spread for 20 seconds on HIGH or until it begins to melt slightly in the tiny glass dish. Stir in the ginger and barbecue sauce after adding them. 2 tbsp of the mixture should be placed in a different, tiny bowl and left aside.

- Brush the chicken with half the sauce after it has finished cooking, then broil for 2 minutes. After turning the drumsticks, coat them with the remaining sauce, and broil them for a further two minutes.

- The drumsticks should be taken out of the broiler, turned over, and brushed with the 2 tablespoons of sauce that were saved for serving.

Nutritional facts:
- Calories 239
- Fat: 5g
- Carbs: 22g
- Protein: 25g
- Sugar: 16g

7.5 Taco-chicken tenders

- Preparation time: 5 minutes
- Cooking time: 7 minutes
- Serving: 4

Ingredients

- 1 pound chicken tenderloins, washed and patted dry
- 4 teaspoons taco seasoning mix
- 2 tablespoons sour cream, fat-free
- 1/2 medium lime

Directions:
- The chicken pieces should have taco seasoning evenly distributed over both sides. Gently push down to help the seasoning stick.

- A big nonstick skillet should be heated up over medium-high heat. Apply nonstick cooking spray to the skillet. Add the chicken, and heat for 2 minutes.

- Turn the chicken gently to preserve as much of the spice as possible, lower the heat to moderate, and cook for 2 minutes. Turn the chicken gently and cook for a further 2 minutes or until the center is no longer pink.

- Serve with 1/2 tbsp of sour cream per dish after removing from heat and equally applying lime juice.

Nutritional facts:
- Calories 144
- Fat: 3g
- Carbs: 2g
- Protein: 25g
- Sugar: 1g

7.6 Rosemary Dijon chicken

- Preparation time: 5 minutes
- Cooking time: 13 minutes
- Serving: 4

Ingredients

- 4 (4 ounce) chicken breasts, boneless and skinless
- 1 tablespoon of Dijon mustard
- 1/4 teaspoon rosemary, dried
- 1 tablespoon olive oil, extra virgin

Directions:

- Set aside after thoroughly blending the olive oil, mustard, and rosemary with a fork in a small bowl.
- Medium heat should be used to heat a medium nonstick skillet. Apply nonstick cooking spray to the skillet. Add the chicken, and heat for 5 minutes.
- After turning the chicken, sprinkle the mustard mixture evenly over each piece. Cook the chicken for 7 mins or until the middle is no longer pink, reducing the heat to medium-low and securely covering the pan.
- Put the chicken on the serving tray and spread the mustard mix over everything, turning the chicken many times to combine the mustard mix with the pan drippings.

Nutritional facts:

- Calories 162
- Fat: 6g
- Carbs: 1g
- Protein: 24g
- Sugar: 0g

7.7 Spinach and goat cheese stuffed chicken

- Preparation time: 30 minutes
- Cooking time: 20 minutes
- Serving: 2

Ingredients

- 1-1/2 cups spinach, chopped
- 1/2 teaspoon pepper, divided
- 2 chicken breasts, boneless skinless
- 1/3 cup (sun-dried) tomatoes, chopped
- 1/4 cup goat cheese, crumbled
- 2 cloves garlic, minced
- 1/2 pound asparagus, trimmed
- 1 tablespoon of olive oil, divided
- 1/2 teaspoon balsamic vinegar (optional)
- 1/4 teaspoon of salt, divided

Directions:

- Set the oven to 400 degrees. Spinach, garlic, goat cheese, sun-dried tomatoes, 1/4 tsp. pepper, and 1/8 tsp. salt should all be combined in a small bowl.
- Each chicken breast's thickest region should have a pocket cut out of it horizontally. Put the spinach mixture inside and fasten it with toothpicks.
- Heat 1 1/2 teaspoons of oil over medium heat in an 8-inch cast-iron or ovenproof pan. Cook the chicken on both sides. Place there; bake for ten minutes.
- In the meantime, combine the asparagus with the final 1-1/2 teaspoons of oil, 1/4 teaspoon of pepper, and 1/8 teaspoon of salt; place in an oven-safe skillet. Bake for a further 10-15 minutes, or until the

chicken thermometer registers 165° and the asparagus is cooked. Add a vinegar drizzle, if desired. Before serving, throw away the toothpicks.

Nutritional facts:

- Calories 347
- Fat: 14g
- Carbs: 6g
- Protein: 39g
- Sugar: 6g

7.8 Lemony au jus chicken

- Preparation time: 20 minutes
- Cooking time: 1 hour 20 minutes
- Serving: 6

Ingredients

- 3 1/2-pound roasting chicken, cleaned and patted dry
- 2 (medium) lemons, quartered
- 3/4 teaspoon powdered garlic
- 1/4 teaspoon of black pepper
- 3/4 teaspoon of poultry seasoning
- 3/4 teaspoon of salt
- 2 cups of water

Directions:

- Set the oven's temperature to 425 degrees.
- Nonstick cooking spray should be sprayed on the broiler rack and pan. Onto the rack, put the chicken. Put the lemon rinds inside the chicken's cavity after equally squeezing the lemons over the bird.
- In a small bowl, mix the garlic powder, poultry

seasoning pepper and salt. Sprinkle equally over the chicken after thoroughly blending. Cook the chicken for 30 minutes after placing it in the oven and adding water through the broiler pan's slits.

- Cook for 50–55 minutes, or till a meat thermometer registers 180 degrees, after reducing the heat to 375 °. The chicken should be taken out of the oven and given 10 minutes to rest on the broiler rack.
- A cutting board should be used for the chicken. Put the pan drippings carefully into a plastic bag with a zipper or a grease separator. To separate the grease, put the drippings in the freezer for ten minutes.
- Remove the oil from the bag or separator, put it onto a microwave-safe glass plate, and heat it for 30 seconds on High. Slice the chicken and serve it with the drippings after removing the skin.

Nutritional facts:

- Calories 265
- Fat: 6g
- Carbs: 1g
- Protein: 25g
- Sugar: 0g

7.9 Crispy chicken in a hot chipotle cream sauce

- Preparation time: 8 minutes
- Cooking time: 14 minutes
- Serving: 4

Ingredients

- 4 (4-ounce) chicken breasts, boneless and skinless
- 1/2 teaspoon salt divided
- 2 tablespoons mayonnaise, reduced-fat
- 6 tablespoons sour cream, fat-free
- 1 1/2 teaspoons total chipotle-chili pepper in adobo sauce, finely chopped
- 1/3 cup of water

Directions:

- Add 1/4 teaspoon salt to the chicken's seasoning. A big nonstick skillet should be heated up over medium-high heat. Cook the chicken for 3 minutes, or until it starts to turn a rich brown, in a skillet coated with nonstick cooking spray.

- Pour water all around the bird after turning it. Cook the chicken for 10 minutes, or until the middle is no longer pink, on medium heat with the cover snugly on.

- In the meantime, combine the mayonnaise, chipotle pepper, sour cream, and 1/4 teaspoon salt in a small bowl.

- Remove the chicken from the skillet and set it on a serving plate. To keep the chicken warm, wrap it in foil.

- Reset the skillet to medium-low heat and put it back on the stove. Add the sour cream mixture and stir it in until everything is well mixed. Stirring continuously; cook for one minute or until well heated. The sauce will separate if it is brought to a boil. To serve, put 2 tbsp. of sauce on each chicken breast.

Nutritional facts:

- Calories 169
- Fat: 5g
- Carbs: 2g
- Protein: 26g
- Sugar: 1g

7.10 White-wine mushroom chicken

- Preparation time: 5 minutes
- Cooking time: 25 minutes
- Serving: 4

Ingredients

- 4 (4-ounce) chicken breasts, boneless and skinless
- 1 cup mushrooms, sliced
- 1/8 teaspoon of black pepper
- 1/4 teaspoon salt, divided
- 1/4 teaspoon rosemary, dried and crushed (optional)
- 2 tablespoons margarine, reduced-fat
- 1/2 cup white wine, dry

Directions:

- A big nonstick skillet should be heated up over medium-high heat. Apply nonstick frying spray to the pan, then put 1/8 tsp. salt and mushrooms. Cook the mushrooms, turning regularly, for 5 min or until the edges start to richly brown. Place the mushrooms on a separate platter and put them aside.

- Add the final 1/8 teaspoon of pepper, salt, and rosemary to the chicken (if using). Reapply nonstick frying spray to the skillet and add the chicken, smooth side down. After 3 minutes, turn the food over and add the wine and mushrooms.

- When the chicken is just no longer pink from the center, turn down the heat, cover firmly, and simmer the mixture for 10 minutes. Only take out the chicken, shake off any leftover mushrooms, and place it on a serving plate. To keep it warm, wrap it in foil.

- The mushroom combination should be heated up to medium-high and boil for two to three minutes or until the majority of the fluid has gone. Take the pan off the heat, add the margarine, and then serve the chicken.

Nutritional facts:

- Calories 173
- Fat: 6g
- Carbs: 3g
- Protein: 25g
- Sugar: 1g

7.11 Tangy chicken and peppers

- Preparation time: 15 minutes
- Cooking time: 42 minutes
- Serving: 4

Ingredients

- 8 chicken drumsticks, washed and patted dry
- 1 (medium) onion, thinly sliced
- 1 large (green) bell pepper, thinly sliced
- 1/8 teaspoon of black pepper
- 1/2 teaspoon salt divided
- 1/4 cup of ketchup
- 1 cup of water

Directions:

- A big nonstick skillet should be heated up over medium-high heat. Spray the skillet with non-stick cooking spray. Add drumsticks in oil, and fry for 8 minutes, turning them over once or twice, until they start to brown. Place the drumsticks on a different platter and put them aside.

- Reapply nonstick cooking spray to the skillet and any leftover pan residue before lowering the heat to medium. Add the onions and peppers, and cook, constantly turning, for 3 mins, or until the edges are just starting to turn gently brown. Add water, pepper, 1/4 tsp salt, and the drumstick and plate juices to the skillet. Bring it to a boil by turning up the heat. Turn down the heat, cover firmly, and let the drumsticks simmer for 30−35 minutes, or until their color is changed from the center.

- Put the drumsticks on a serving dish with a rim or a shallow pasta bowl. To the pepper mix in the skillet, add 1/4 teaspoon salt and the ketchup. The mixture should boil for 1 min or until it is decreased to 2 cups after increasing the heat to high.

- The drumsticks should be covered and left to stand in the pepper mixture for five minutes to let the flavors meld

Nutritional facts:

- Calories 268
- Fat: 8g
- Carbs: 10g
- Protein: 38g
- Sugar: 4g

7.12 Turkey breast chili

- Preparation time: 20 minutes
- Cooking time: 1 hour 20 minutes
- Serving: 12

Ingredients

- 6-pound (bone-in) turkey breast, frozen and thawed
- 1 1/2 teaspoons of chili powder
- 3/4 teaspoon sage, dried
- 1/2 teaspoon of black pepper
- 1/2 teaspoon rosemary, dried
- 3/4 teaspoon salt, divided
- 2/3 cup of cold water

Directions:

- Set the oven's temperature to 325.
- In a small bowl, combine the rosemary, sage, chili powder, pepper, and 1/2 tsp salt. Stir until thoroughly combined. By placing your fingertips in between the turkey's meat and the skin, you can loosen the skin on the bird's breast (do not remove the skin). Rub the turkey's inner meat with the chili mixture.
- The turkey should be baked for 1 hour and 45 minutes, or till a meat thermometer reads 165 degrees, in a 13 x 9-inch baking pan and rack coated with nonstick cooking spray. On a chopping board, place the turkey, and let it stand for 20 minutes.
- In the meantime, combine the pan drippings with the remaining 1/4 tsp and water salt by stirring them together. Put the pan drippings carefully into a zippered plastic bag or a grease separator. To separate the grease, put the drippings in the freezer for ten minutes.
- Grease should be removed from the bag or separator, poured onto a glass tray, and heated on high flame for 30 sec in the microwave. Sliced turkey is served with the drippings, and the skin is removed.

Nutritional facts:

- Calories 176
- Fat: 1g
- Carbs: 0g
- Protein: 39g
- Sugar: 0g

7.13 Hoisin chicken

- Preparation time: 10 minutes
- Cooking time: 8 minutes
- Serving: 4

Ingredients

- 1 pound chicken breasts, slices / strips
- 3 tablespoons of hoisin sauce
- 3 tablespoons of orange juice
- 1 teaspoon of orange zest

Directions:

- Hoisin sauce, orange juice, and zest are combined in a small bowl and let stand.
- Medium-high heat should be used to heat a medium nonstick skillet. Cook the chicken in the skillet for 6-7 minutes, or until it just starts to turn light brown, after spraying it with nonstick cooking spray. When stir-frying, use 2 utensils to stir.
- The chicken should be put on a serving plate. Cook for 15 seconds while constantly swirling the hoisin mixture in the skillet. Overlapping the chicken with a spoon.

Nutritional facts:

- Calories 152
- Fat: 3g
- Carbs: 5g
- Protein: 25g
- Sugar: 5g

7.14 Skillet chicken and spinach pasta

- Preparation time: 10 minutes
- Cooking time: 25 minutes
- Serving: 4

Ingredients

- 1 pound chicken breast cut into (bite-size) pieces
- 8 ounces of penne pasta, gluten-free
- ½ teaspoon of salt
- 4 garlic cloves, minced
- 2 tablespoons olive oil, extra-virgin
- ¼ teaspoon pepper, ground
- ½ cup white wine, dry
- 10 cups spinach, chopped fresh
- 1 lemon zest and juice
- 4 tablespoons Parmesan cheese, grated and divided

Directions:

- As directed on the package, cook the pasta. Drain then set apart.
- Oil should be heated in a big, high-sided skillet in the meantime over medium-high heat. Cook, stirring regularly, for 5 to 7 minutes, until chicken is just cooked through. Add chicken, salt, and pepper. Add the garlic and stir-fry for approximately a minute or until fragrant. Add wine, lemon juice, and zest; simmer after stirring. Get rid of the heat. Add cooked pasta and spinach to the mixture. As soon as the spinach has just begun to wilt, cover and leave. Distribute among 4 dishes and sprinkle 1 tablespoon Parmesan cheese over each portion.

Nutritional facts:

- Calories 335
- Fat: 12g
- Carbs: 24g
- Protein: 28g
- Sugar: 1g

CHAPTER 8: SNACKS AND SIDES

8.1 Lemony shrimp

- o Preparation time: 5 minutes
- o Cooking time: 10 minutes
- o Serving: 8

Ingredients

- o 12 ounces (medium) shrimp, frozen and thawed
- o 1 teaspoon of lemon zest
- o 2 tablespoons margarine, reduced-fat
- o 3 tablespoons of lemon juice
- o 2 tablespoons of Worcestershire sauce
- o 1 tablespoon fresh parsley, finely chopped (optional)

Directions

- o A big nonstick skillet should be heated up over medium heat. To the skillet, add the shrimp, lemon juice, Worcestershire sauce, and lemon zest. Stirring constantly, cook the shrimp for 5 min or until the center is opaque.
- o The shrimp should be taken out with a slotted spoon and placed in a serving bowl. Margarine should be added, warmed to a boil, and then continuously stirred for 2 mins or until the mixture measures 1/4 cup.
- o If desired, drizzle the sauce on the shrimp and garnish with parsley. Use wooden toothpicks when serving.

Nutritional facts:

- o Calories 47
- o Fat: 2g
- o Carbs: 1g
- o Protein: 7g
- o Sugar: 1g

8.2 Plantain chips (Air fryer)

- o Preparation time: 10 minutes
- o Cooking time: 10 minutes
- o Serving: 2

Ingredients

- o 1 green-plantain
- o 1 pinch of salt
- o Avocado-oil spray

Directions

- o Achieve a 350°F air fryer temperature (175 degrees C).
- o Plantain should be cut in half, with the skin merely being scored along the side. Plantain should be peeled and sliced in half. Utilizing a vegetable peeler, cut into strips.
- o Spray avocado oil on the air fryer basket. Plantain strips should not touch as they are placed in the basket. Apply oil on the top of the plantain slices.
- o Cook for 7 - 9 mins in the prepared air fryer. Using tongs, flip each strip and continue frying for a further 3 to 5 minutes or until crisp. Salt should be added right away.

Nutritional facts:

- o Calories 109
- o Fat: 0g

- o Carbs: 29g
- o Protein: 1g
- o Sugar: 13g

8.3 Air-fry radishes

- o Preparation time: 5 minutes
- o Cooking time: 15 minutes
- o Serving: 6

Ingredients

- o 3 tablespoons of olive oil
- o 6 cups radishes, quartered
- o 1 teaspoon oregano, dried
- o 1/8 teaspoon of pepper
- o 1/4 teaspoon of salt

Directions

- o Preheat the air fryer to 375°F. Toss the remaining ingredients with the radishes. Put the radishes in the air fryer basket on the oiled tray. Cook for 12 to 15 minutes, stirring periodically, until crisp-tender.

Nutritional facts:

- o Calories 88
- o Fat: 7g
- o Carbs: 6g
- o Protein: 1g

Sugar: 3g

8.5 Lemon and herb cauliflower (Air-fryer)

- o Preparation time: 10 minutes
- o Cooking time: 10 minutes
- o Serving: 4

Ingredients

- o 4 tablespoons of olive oil, divided
- o 6 cups cauliflower head, florets
- o 1/4 cup parsley, minced fresh
- o 1 tablespoon thyme, minced fresh
- o 1 tablespoon rosemary, minced fresh
- o 1 teaspoon lemon zest, grated
- o 2 tablespoons of lemon juice
- o 1/4 teaspoon red pepper flakes, crushed
- o 1/2 teaspoon of salt

Directions

- o Preheat the air fryer to 350°F. Combine 2 tbsp of olive oil and cauliflower in a large bowl, and toss to coat. Cauliflower should be placed on a tray in the air fryer basket in batches and in single layers. Cook for 8 to 10 mins, stirring halfway through, or until the edges are browned, and the florets are soft. Add the remaining ingredients and 2 tablespoons of oil to a small bowl. Place the cauliflower in a sizable bowl, drizzle with the herb mixture, and combine.

Nutritional facts:

- o Calories 161
- o Fat: 14g
- o Carbs: 8g
- o Protein: 3g
- o Sugar: 3g

8.6 Kale cheesy chips

- o Preparation time: 5 minutes
- o Cooking time: 45 minutes

- o Serving: 6

Ingredients

- o 2 tablespoons olive oil, extra virgin
- o ⅓ teaspoon of salt
- o ½ cup of nutritional yeast
- o 1 bunch of curly kale, torn

Directions

- o Preheat the oven to 200°F (95 degrees C).
- o In a large dish, toss the kale with the salt and nutritional yeast before adding the olive oil. To coat the kale, stir it with your hands.
- o Kale is spread out on baking sheets.
- o Bake in pre - a heated oven till kale starts to get lightly crisp; then, flip the chips over and rotate the racks, roasting until the kale is thoroughly crisp, another 45 to 60 minutes. Maintain a watchful eye on them to ensure they wouldn't burn; if you see that specific chips are ready considerably sooner than others, remove them.

Nutritional facts:

- o Calories 111
- o Fat: 6g
- o Carbs: 11g
- o Protein: 8g
- o Sugar: 1g

8.7 Homemade guacamole

- o Preparation time: 10 minutes
- o Cooking time: 0 minutes
- o Serving: 2cups

Ingredients

- o 3 medium avocados, cubed
- o 1/4 - 1/2 teaspoon of salt
- o 1 clove garlic, minced
- o 1 - 2 tablespoons lime juice
- o 1 small onion, thinly chopped
- o 1 tablespoon fresh cilantro, minced
- o 1/4 cup of mayonnaise, optional
- o 2 (medium) tomatoes, chopped (optional)

Directions

- o Avocados are mashed with salt and garlic. Add the other ingredients and, if you like, the tomatoes and mayonnaise.

Nutritional facts:

- o Calories 90
- o Fat: 8g
- o Carbs: 1g
- o Protein: 6g
- o Sugar: 1g

8.8 Rosemary walnuts

- o Preparation time: 10 minutes
- o Cooking time: 10 minutes
- o Serving: 2 cups

Ingredients

- o 2 cups walnut halves
- o 2 teaspoons rosemary, dried and crushed
- o 1/4 - 1/2 teaspoon of cayenne pepper
- o 1/2 teaspoon of kosher salt

- o Cooking spray

Directions

- o Put the walnuts in a little bowl. Spray some frying spray on. Seasonings added, toss to coat. Place on a baking sheet in a single layer.

- o Bake for 10 minutes at 350°. Warm up before serving or let cool completely before storing in an airtight container.

Nutritional facts:

- o Calories 166
- o Fat: 17g
- o Carbs: 4g
- o Protein: 4g
- o Sugar: 1g

8.9 Lime blueberries

- o Preparation time: 5 minutes
- o Cooking time: 0 minutes
- o Serving: 4

Ingredients

- o 2 cups unsweetened blueberries, frozen and partially thawed
- o 1 1/2 tablespoons of lime juice
- o 1/4 cup grape juice concentrate, frozen

Directions

- o In a medium bowl, combine all the ingredients and toss gently.
- o To have the best flavor and texture, serve right away.

Nutritional facts:

- o Calories 83

- o Fat: 0g
- o Carbs: 20g
- o Protein: 0g
- o Sugar: 17g

8.10 Creamy fruit dip

- o Preparation time: 5 minutes
- o Cooking time: 0 minutes
- o Serving: 4

Ingredients

- o 1/4 cup whipped topping, fat-free
- o 1/3 cup vanilla yogurt, fat-free
- o 2 tablespoons apricot (all-fruit) Spread
- o 1 medium apple, sliced
- o 1 cups strawberries, whole

Directions

- o Mix the yogurt, fruit, and whipped topping spread thoroughly in a small bowl.
- o Serve alongside fruit.

Nutritional facts:

- o Calories 56
- o Fat: 0g
- o Carbs: 13g
- o Protein: 9g
- o Sugar: 1g

8.11 Cheese pears

- o Preparation time: 5 minutes
- o Cooking time: 0 minutes
- o Serving: 4

Ingredients

- o 2 ounces cream cheese, fat-free
- o 2 medium pears, cored, halved, and cut into 20 slices
- o 1/4 cup bleu cheese, crumbled

Directions

- o The cheeses should be heated in a small bowl for 10 seconds on HIGH to soften. When blending, use a rubber spatula.
- o Each pear slice should have 3/4 teaspoon of cheese on top.
- o Toss the pear slices with a pineapple, a tbsp of orange, or lemon juice to prevent them from becoming brown. Shake off any extra moisture before adding cheese to them.

Nutritional facts:

- o Calories 88
- o Fat: 2g
- o Carbs: 14g
- o Protein: 4g
- o Sugar: 9g

8.12 Crackers and basil spread

- o Preparation time: 5 minutes
- o Cooking time: 0 minutes
- o Serving: 4

Ingredients

- o 1/4 cup fresh basil, finely chopped
- o 2 ounces herb and garlic cream cheese, reduced-fat
- o 12 water crackers, fat-free

Directions

- o In a small bowl, combine the basil and cream cheese and stir until well combined.
- o On each cracker, spread 1 teaspoon of the sauce.

Nutritional facts:

- o Calories 63
- o Fat: 2g
- o Carbs: 8g
- o Protein: 3g
- o Sugar: 0g

8.13 Carrots with spicy cream dip

- o Preparation time: 5 minutes
- o Cooking time: 0 minutes
- o Serving: 4

Ingredients

- o 1/3 cup sour cream, fat-free
- o 3/4 teaspoon hot-pepper sauce
- o 3 tablespoons cream cheese, reduced-fat
- o 48 (baby) carrots
- o 1/4 teaspoon salt

Directions

- o Stir together the cream cheese, pepper sauce, sour cream, and salt until completely combined.
- o Allow it to rest for a minimum of 10 min to let flavors meld and slightly mellow. Accompanied by carrots.

Nutritional facts:

- o Calories 73
- o Fat: 2g
- o Carbs: 10g

- o Protein: 3g
- o Sugar: 5g

8.14 Sweet peanut Buttery dip

- o Preparation time: 5 minutes
- o Cooking time: 0 minutes
- o Serving: 4

Ingredients

- o 2 (medium) bananas, sliced
- o 1/3 cup vanilla yogurt, fat-free
- o 2 teaspoons dark-brown sugar
- o 2 tablespoons peanut butter, reduced-fat

Directions

- o Stir the peanut butter, yogurt, and brown sugar in a bowl with a whisk or fork until well combined.
- o If desired, serve with slices of banana and wooden toothpicks.

Nutritional facts:

- o Calories 73
- o Fat: 2g
- o Carbs: 10g
- o Protein: 3g
- o Sugar: 5g

8.15 Grilled corn

- o Preparation time: 15 minutes
- o Cooking time: 15 minutes
- o Serving: 6

Ingredients

- o 6 medium ears-sweet corn
- o 1 tablespoon of lime juice

- o 1/4 cup Parmesan cheese, grated
- o 1/2 teaspoon of chili powder
- o 1/8 teaspoon of pepper
- o 1/4 teaspoon of salt
- o 1/2 cup of sour cream

Directions

- o To remove the silk, carefully peel aside the corn husks up to 1 inch from the bottom. Put corn back in its husks and tie it up with kitchen twine. Corn husks should be moistened by rinsing in water. Covered, grill corn for 20–25 minutes at medium heat, turning frequently or until tender.
- o Blend the remaining ingredients in a small bowl. Remove the string from the corn and the husks. Apply the sour cream mixture to the corn.

Nutritional facts:

- o Calories 143
- o Fat: 6g
- o Carbs: 20g
- o Protein: 5g
- o Sugar: 7g

8.16 Marinated mushrooms

- o Preparation time: 5 minutes
- o Cooking time: 8 minutes
- o Serving: 4

Ingredients

- o 8 ounces medium mushrooms, whole
- o 1 teaspoon olive oil, extra virgin
- o 2 tablespoons lite-soy sauce
- o 2 tablespoons of lime juice

- o 2 tablespoons parsley, chopped fresh (optional)

Directions

- o Put the oil, lime juice, soy sauce, and mushrooms in a sizable plastic zippered bag. Shake the bag thoroughly after sealing it. Pause for 30 minutes, and in the interim, warm up the broiler.

- o In an 8-inch baking dish or pie pan, place the mushroom mixture with marinade) and broil it 4 inches distant from the source of heat for 8 minutes or till the mushrooms start to brown, tossing often.

- o Serve with marinade and wooden toothpicks.

Nutritional facts:

- o Calories 29

- o Fat: 1g

- o Carbs: 4g

- o Protein: 2g

- o Sugar: 1g

CHAPTER 9: FISHES AND SEAFOOD

- o Preparation time: 5 minutes
- o Cooking time: 6 minutes
- o Serving: 4

Ingredients

- o 4 (4-ounce) tuna steaks, washed and patted dry
- o 1/4 cup mayonnaise, reduced-fat
- o 1/4 teaspoon of black pepper
- o 1/2 teaspoon garlic, minced
- o 1/4 cup sour cream, fat-free
- o 1/2 teaspoon salt divided

Directions

- o Preheat the grill or the broiler over high heat.
- o In a small bowl, combine the sour cream, garlic, mayonnaise, and 1/4 tsp salt.
- o Over the steaks, season with 1/4 tsp each of pepper and salt. Spray some nonstick cooking spray on the broiler or grill rack and pan. The steaks should be grilled or broiled for three minutes on each side or until done to preference.
- o Along with the steaks, serve the sauce.

Nutritional facts:

- o Calories 218
- o Fat: 10g
- o Carbs: 2g
- o Protein: 27g
- o Sugar: 1g

- o Preparation time: 5 minutes
- o Cooking time: 20 minutes
- o Serving: 4

Ingredients

- o 4 tilapia fillets
- o 1 tablespoon of butter
- o 1/4 teaspoon of pepper
- o 1 (medium)tomato, finely sliced
- o 1/4 teaspoon of salt

Topping:

- o 2 tablespoons of lemon juice
- o 1/4 cup walnuts, chopped
- o 1-1/2 teaspoons of butter, melted
- o 1/2 cup breadcrumbs

Directions

- o Fillets should be salted and peppered. In a large skillet sprayed with cooking oil, fry the fillets in butter on medium-high heat for two to three minutes per side until lightly browned.
- o Place the fish on a baking sheet or broiler pan, then add the tomato.
- o Spoon the tomato slices on top after combining the topping ingredients.
- o Broil 3-4 inches from the fire for 2-3 minutes, or until the topping is slightly browned and the fish begins to flake readily with a fork.

Nutritional facts:

- Calories 202
- Fat, 10g
- Carbs: 6g
- Protein: 23g
- Sugar: 2g

9.3 Lemony baked cod

- Preparation time: 5 minutes
- Cooking time: 20 minutes
- Serving: 4

Ingredients

- 4 cod fillets
- 3 tablespoons parsley, minced fresh
- 1 tablespoon lemon zest, grated
- 2 tablespoons of lemon juice
- 1 tablespoon of olive oil
- 1/8 teaspoon of pepper
- 1/4 teaspoon of salt
- 2 (green) onions, chopped
- 2 cloves garlic, minced

Directions

- Set the oven to 400 degrees. Mix the initial 7 ingredients in a small bowl. Cod should be placed in an 11x7-inch baking dish that has not been buttered. Add some green onions on top. Bake, covered, for 10-15 minutes or until fish flakes easily.

Nutritional facts:

- Calories 161
- Fat: 4g
- Carbs: 2g
- Protein: 27g

- Sugar: 0g

9.4 Flounder topped with cucumber

- Preparation time: 7 minutes
- Cooking time: 12-15 minutes
- Serving: 4

Ingredients

- 4 (4-ounce) flounder filets, rinsed and patted dry
- 1/2 (medium) cucumber, finely chopped
- 1/2 teaspoon of lime zest
- 2 tablespoons mayonnaise, reduced-fat
- 1/4 teaspoon of salt
- 1 tablespoon of lime juice
- Lime wedges (optional)
- 1/4 teaspoon of black pepper

Directions

- Set the oven's temperature to 400.
- Cooking spray and foil are used to line a baking pan. The fillets should be spaced about two inches apart on the foil. Apply nonstick cooking spray to the fillets, then equally sprinkle pepper over them. Bake for 12 to 15 minutes or until the fillets are opaque throughout.
- In the meantime, combine the lime zest, juice, mayonnaise, and salt in a small bowl and whisk to combine.
- Place the fillets on a serving plate, top with sauce, and serve with additional lime wedges on the side, if preferred.

Nutritional facts:

- Calories 130
- Fat: 4g
- Carbs: 1g
- Protein: 22g
- Sugar: 1g

9.5 Saucy cajun fish

- Preparation time: 10 minutes
- Cooking time: 12-15 minutes
- Serving: 4

Ingredients

- 4 (4-ounce) tilapia filets, washed and patted dry
- 2 tablespoons margarine, reduced-fat
- 14 .5-ounce can tomatoes stewed with Cajun seasonings, drained
- 2 tablespoons parsley, chopped fresh (optional)
- 1/2 teaspoon of seafood seasoning

Directions

- Set the oven's temperature to 400.
- The fish fillets should be spaced about 2 inches apart on the broiler rack, and the seafood seasoning should be distributed equally over them.
- The tomatoes should be blended just till smooth. In a small dish, reserve 1/4 cup of mixture.
- Each fillet should have the remaining tomatoes distributed evenly over the top. Bake the fillets for 12 to 15 minutes or until the center is opaque.
- In the meantime, combine the saved 1/4 cup of tomato mixture with the margarine and microwave it on HIGH for 20 seconds or till the mixture is barely melted. Stir well to combine.
- Place the fillets on a serving tray, top each with a dollop of the tomato-margarine mixture, and top with optional parsley.

Nutritional facts:

- Calories 163
- Fat: 5g
- Carbs: 6g
- Protein: 23g
- Sugar: 4g

9.6 Fish tacos (Air-fryer)

- Preparation time: 5 minutes
- Cooking time: 30 minutes
- Serving: 4

Ingredients

- 1 pound (mahi-mahi) fillets, cut into (2- to 3-inch) strip
- 2 cups green cabbage, shredded
- ¼ cup fresh cilantro, coarsely chopped
- 1 (large) avocado
- 5 tablespoons of lime juice divided
- 1 scallion, finely sliced
- 1 tablespoon of avocado oil
- 2 tablespoons of sour cream
- 1 small garlic clove, grated
- 1 (large) egg white
- ¼ teaspoon of salt
- ⅓ cup breadcrumbs, whole-wheat

- ○ 8 corn (medium) tomato, chopped
- ○ 1 tablespoon of chili powder
- ○ Avocado oil-cooking spray

Directions

- ○ In a medium bowl, combine the cilantro, cabbage, scallion, 2 tbsp lime juice, and avocado oil.

- ○ Avocados should be cut in half lengthwise, and the pulp should be placed in the bowl of a small food processor using a spoon. Process the remaining 3 tbsp of lime juice, garlic, salt, sour cream, and sour cream for about 30 seconds or until smooth. (Or you can use a fork to mash until the consistency you want is achieved.) Place aside.

- ○ Preheat the air fryer to 400oF. In a shallow dish, add the egg white; whisk until foamy. In a different shallow dish, mix chili powder and breadcrumbs. Utilizing a paper towel, dry the fish. Put the fish in egg white mixture to coat. Then, dredge the fish in the bread-crumb mix and press firmly to coat, letting excess fall off.

- ○ Place the fish in the frying basket in an even layer; if necessary, work in batches. Coat the fish thoroughly with cooking spray. Cook for about 3 minutes or until brown and crispy on one side. Cook the salmon until it is crisp and flakes readily, about 3 mins after flipping it. Fish should be flaked into bite-sized pieces. Fish, cabbage slaw (1/4 cup per), avocado crème (about 1 tbsp per), and tomato are evenly distributed on top of each tortilla. If preferred, serve with lime wedges.

Nutritional facts:

- ○ Calories 377
- ○ Fat: 15g
- ○ Carbs: 36g
- ○ Protein: 27g
- ○ Sugar: 3g

9.7 Caper cream tilapia

- ○ Preparation time: 6 minutes
- ○ Cooking time: 6 minutes
- ○ Serving: 4

Ingredients

- ○ 4 (4-ounce) tilapia filets, washed and patted dry
- ○ 1 tablespoon of capers, drained
- ○ 1/4 cup sour cream, reduced-fat
- ○ 1/4 teaspoon of black pepper
- ○ 1/4 teaspoon of salt, divided
- ○ 1 (medium) lemon, quartered

Directions

- ○ To mash the capers, you can use the back of a fork or a spoon. Mix the sour cream with the 1/8 tsp salt and capers.

- ○ Heat up a sizable nonstick skillet on medium heat. Spray some nonstick cooking spray on the skillet. Each fillet should have 1/8 teaspoon salt and black pepper uniformly distributed on one side. Cook for 3 minutes, turn, and cook for an additional two to three minutes or until the salmon is opaque throughout.

- Place the fillets on a serving tray, drizzle 1 spoonful of sour cream over each, then squeeze 1 tbsp lemon juice equally overall.

Nutritional facts:

- Calories 135
- Fat: 4g
- Carbs: 2g
- Protein: 23g
- Sugar: 1g

9.8 White-wine reduction scallops

- Preparation time: 5 minutes
- Cooking time: 25 minutes
- Serving: 8

Ingredients

- 2 pounds of sea scallops
- 2 tablespoons of olive oil
- 1 teaspoon of salt
- 1/4 teaspoon of pepper

White-wine reduction:

- 1/4 cup onion, finely chopped
- 1/2 cup white wine or chicken broth
- 1 teaspoon oregano, dried
- 1 clove garlic, minced
- 1 teaspoon of Dijon mustard
- 3 tablespoons butter, cubed
- 1/3 cup of orange juice

Directions

- Scallops should be salted and peppered. Scallops should be cooked in oil in a big skillet until opaque and firm. Get rid of it and keep warm.

- Pour wine into the skillet while stirring to remove any browned particles. Add the onion, orange juice, mustard, oregano, and garlic to the mixture. Bring to a boil and cook, constantly stirring, till reduced by half, about 2-3 minutes. Butter is added after the heat source has been turned off. Serve alongside scallops.

Nutritional facts:

- Calories 181
- Fat: 9g
- Carbs: 5g
- Protein: 19g
- Sugar: 1g

9.9 Ahi-tuna poke

- Preparation time: 5 minutes
- Cooking time: 10 minutes
- Serving: 2

Ingredients

- ½ pound ahi-tuna steaks
- 1 avocado, diced
- 2 tablespoons soy sauce, low-sodium
- 1 tablespoon chili-garlic sauce
- 1 tablespoon of sesame oil
- 2 sprigs of green onions, finely chopped
- 1 tablespoon of sesame seeds divided

Directions

- Ahi tuna should be rinsed before being dried with paper towels to eliminate extra moisture. Create bite-sized chunks of raw tuna.

- Mix the soy sauce, chopped green onions, sesame oil, garlic chili sauce, and ½ of the sesame seeds in a small bowl.

- When the tuna is thoroughly coated, drizzle the soy-sauce mix on the ahi cubes and swirl to combine. To let the flavors mingle, place in the refrigerator for 10–20 minutes or up to 24 hours.

- Mix the ahi fish cubes with the combination of sesame oil until all piece of tuna is evenly coated. After that, you can chill it for a minimum of 10 to 20 minutes to allow the flavors to mingle, but it's not necessary.

- Before serving, carefully fold the avocado, which has been cut into small cubes, into the tuna poke.

- Serve with the remaining sesame seeds as a garnish.

Nutritional facts:

- Calories 433
- Fat: 29g
- Carbs: 13g
- Protein: 31g
- Sugar: 3g

9.10 Nicoise tuna salad

- Preparation time: 10 minutes
- Cooking time: 5 minutes
- Serving: 1

Ingredients

- 4 ounces ahi-tuna steak
- ½ red-bell pepper
- 2 ounces green beans
- 2 cup baby spinach
- 1½ ounces broccoli
- 1 radish
- 1 egg, whole
- 1 teaspoon of olive oil
- 1 tablespoon parsley
- 3½ ounces cucumber
- 1 teaspoon of balsamic vinegar
- ½ teaspoon of pepper
- ½ teaspoon of Dijon mustard
- 3 (large) black olives

Directions

- The egg should be boiled and then let to cool.

- Set aside after steaming the broccoli and beans. It only takes a few seconds in the microwave for two to three minutes or three minutes in a saucepan of boiling water.

- In a pan, heat a small amount of oil over high heat. The tuna should be peppered all over before being added to the pan and seared for 2 minutes per side.

- Place the spinach in the salad bowl or on the dish.

- Cut the cucumber, egg, and bell pepper into bite-sized pieces. Add to the spinach's top.

- Slice the radish and combine it with the beans, broccoli, and olives. Add to the spinach salad on top.

- Add the sliced tuna to the salad.

- o Mix the salt, olive oil, mustard, balsamic vinegar, and pepper together.
- o Add the chopped parsley to the vinaigrette.
- o Pour the vinaigrette on the salad.

Nutritional facts:

- o Calories 405
- o Fat: 13g
- o Carbs: 18g
- o Protein: 39g
- o Sugar: 8g

9.11 Celery parsley snapper fillet

- o Preparation time: 5 minutes
- o Cooking time: 20 minutes
- o Serving: 4

Ingredients

- o 4 snapper fillets, wild-caught
- o 8 sticks of celery
- o ½ tablespoon of honey
- o ½ bunch of flat parsley
- o 1 tablespoon of tahini
- o 3 tablespoons of olive oil
- o 1 lemon, juice
- o Pepper
- o Sea salt

Directions

- o Set the oven to 350°F (175C).
- o A baking sheet should be lightly greased with olive oil.
- o Place fish fillets with the skin side down on a baking sheet and liberally season with sea salt and black pepper.
- o Depending on the thickness, bake for roughly 15 to 18 minutes.
- o Wash the celery and cut off the ends and leaves while the fish cooks. Cut into thin sticks that are 1" long and 1/8" thick, then place in a bowl.
- o Parsley should be cleaned and de-stalked before being dried and chopped coarsely. Add to the celery-filled bowl.
- o Shake the ingredients in a sealable container (like a mason jar) to thoroughly blend the olive oil, tahini, lemon juice, and honey.
- o When the fish is done, take it out of the oven and serve it with a tahini sauce and celery-parsley salad. If desired, add one more squeeze of lemon on top.

Nutritional facts:

- o Calories 313
- o Fat: 15g
- o Carbs: 6g
- o Protein: 35g
- o Sugar: 3.5g

CHAPTER 10: DESSERT

10.1 Protein cheesecake (Low carb)

- o Preparation time: 10 minutes
- o Cooking time: 50 minutes
- o Serving: 2

Ingredients

- o 2 egg whites
- o 8.5 ounces cottage cheese, low fat
- o 1 tablespoon of stevia
- o 1 scoop of vanilla protein powder
- o 1 teaspoon of vanilla extract
- o Water
- o 1 serving Strawberry Jell-O, sugar-free

Directions

- o Oven: 325 degrees Fahrenheit (160 C).
- o In accordance with the directions on the package, prepare the Jell-O, then put it in the freezer.
- o The consistency should be smooth after blending egg whites and cottage cheese.
- o The protein powder, vanilla extract, and Stevia should be whisked into the combined mixture once it has been poured into a bowl.
- o Bake the batter for 25 minutes after pouring it into a little nonstick pan.
- o Switch off the oven and keep the cake in there to cool. Remove the cheesecake from the oven after it has cooled.
- o Pour the Jell-O over the cheesecake once it is nearly set.
- o Prior to consumption, let the cake rest in the refrigerator for at least 10 to 12 hours.

Nutritional facts:

- o Calories 165
- o Fat: 0.5g
- o Carbs: 6g
- o Protein: 32g
- o Sugar: 3.5g

10.2 Lemonade strawberry popsicles

- o Preparation time: 5 minutes
- o Cooking time: 0 minutes
- o Serving: 6

Ingredients

- o ¼ cup oats, old-fashioned
- o 4 ounces of lemon juice
- o 1½ pounds strawberries
- o 4 ounces cottage cheese, low fat
- o 5 drops of liquid Stevia

Directions

- o In a powerful blender or food processor, pulse the oats until they are powdered.
- o Then process it until smooth after including the cottage cheese, strawberries, lemon juice, and stevia. If required, turn off the blender and use a spatula to push the items down. Add no liquids at all!

- Place the mixture into six Popsicle molds and freeze for at least three hours until solid.

Nutritional facts:

- Calories 73
- Fat: 0.5g
- Carbs: 14g
- Protein: 3g
- Sugar: 8g

10.3 Raspberry pumpkin muffins

- Preparation time: 15 minutes
- Cooking time: 25 minutes
- Serving: 12

Ingredients

- 1 cup of pumpkin puree
- 3/4 cup almond flour, blanched
- 1/2 cup of coconut flour
- 1 tablespoon of baking powder
- 3 tablespoon arrowroot or tapioca starch
- 1 tablespoon of cinnamon
- 1/4 teaspoon salt
- 1/8 teaspoon nutmeg
- 1/2 cup stevia
- 4 egg-yolks
- 4 egg -whites
- 1 1/2 teaspoons of vanilla extract
- 1 1/2 cups raspberries, frozen
- 1/2 cup f coconut oil, melted
- 10 drops of liquid stevia

Directions

- Set your oven's temperature to 350°F (177°C) and insert muffin papers into each of the 12 muffin cups.
- The coconut flour, nutmeg, stevia, almond flour, baking powder, tapioca starch, cinnamon, and sea salt should all be thoroughly combined in a big basin.
- Until everything is thoroughly combined, stir in the egg yolks (save the egg whites for the following step), coconut oil, pumpkin puree, stevia drops, and vanilla.
- The egg whites should be beaten until firm white peaks form in a separate basin.
- In the muffin batter, combine the frozen raspberries and egg whites.
- Advice: Be careful not to overmix the mixture at this point because doing so will make the muffins dense. Simply use a spatula or spoon to gently mix the raspberry egg whites into the batter.
- Fill the muffin papers with the batter, then level the tops. The muffin mixture should come just to the upper edge of the paper cups. Because these muffins don't rise very high, fill the muffin papers to the brim.
- The muffins should bake for 25 minutes. A toothpick should be put into the muffins, which will be lightly browned on top. After five minutes, remove the muffins from the muffin tin and let them cool fully on a cooling rack.

Nutritional facts:

- o Calories 217
- o Fat: 14g
- o Carbs: 14g
- o Protein: 5g
- o Sugar: 2g

10.4 Pumpkin–banana snack cake

- o Preparation time: 5 minutes
- o Cooking time: 20 minutes
- o Serving: 8

Ingredients

- o 1/2 can (15-ounce) solid pumpkin (not pumpkin pie) mix
- o 4 teaspoons of cinnamon sugar
- o 6 boxes (0.4-ounce) banana-nut muffin mix
- o 1/2 cup of water

Directions

- o Set the oven's temperature to 400.
- o In a medium bowl, combine the water and pumpkin with a fork and whisk until completely combined. Stir in the muffin mix after adding it (It will be lumpy batter). Avoid overmixing.
- o Apply a thin layer of nonstick cooking spray to an 8 x 8-inch baking pan and pour the batter. Bake for 20 to 22 minutes or until nearly no batter remains on a wooden toothpick.
- o Place the cake on the wire rack to rest for 15 minutes while the flavors develop. When serving, top each piece with 1/2 teaspoon of cinnamon sugar.

Nutritional facts:

- o Calories 111

- o Fat: 3g
- o Carbs: 21g
- o Protein: 2g
- o Sugar: 10g

10.5 Berry pie bowl

- o Preparation time: 20 minutes
- o Cooking time: 4 minutes
- o Serving: 15

Ingredients

- o 2 pounds (unsweetened) blackberries, frozen
- o 1 refrigerated pie crust, reduced-fat
- o 4 cups frozen yogurt or vanilla ice cream
- o 10-ounce jar of raspberry (all-fruit) spread

Directions

- o Set the oven's temperature to 475.
- o Take the pie crust out of the packaging and allow it to stand as instructed. The pie crust should be spread out on a cutting board. Cut 10 rounds with a 3-inch biscuit cutter. A ball of dough should be formed, and it should then be rolled out to the same thickness. Remove more rounds. You'll have 15 rounds after rolling and chopping one more time.
- o Place the rounds on a large baking sheet, brush the baking sheet with non-stick cooking spray, and bake for 4 minutes or till the rounds are just beginning to turn brown. The rounds should be placed on a cooling rack to cool properly when the baking sheet has been taken out of the oven.
- o In the meantime, heat a sizable skillet over medium-high heat. Melt the

fruit spread by adding it and stirring. Bring to a boil after adding the blackberries. Cook for 4 minutes, stirring gently and regularly, till the berries are well-cooked and slightly softened.

- The berries should cool completely after being removed from the fire and allowed to stand for two hours. The mixture can thicken a little bit, and the flavors can mellow as a result. (You could wrap the mixture in plastic and put it in the fridge. After refrigerating, the mixture will become quite thick.)

- A pie round should be placed in the base of each ramekin or dessert bowl before 1/4 cup of berry mix is added on top. To serve this dish warm, cover the dishes with plastic and microwave them for 15–20 seconds on high power. 1/4 cup of circular ice cream is added to each serving.

Nutritional facts:

- Calories 184
- Fat: 4g
- Carbs: 37g
- Protein: 3g
- Sugar: 16g

10.6 Strawberries in double-rich cream

- Preparation time: 10 minutes
- Cooking time: 0 minutes
- Serving: 4

Ingredients

- 6-ounce jar vanilla yogurt, fat-free

- 1-pint strawberries, quartered
- 1 1/2 ounces (tub-style) cream cheese, reduced-fat
- 1 cup whipped topping, fat-free

Directions

- Blend the cream cheese and yoghurt in a blender until they are thoroughly combined.

- The liquid should be poured into a bowl along with the whipping topping and strawberries. Gently swirl to combine.

- Serve right away or chill for up to eight hours covered in plastic wrap.

Nutritional facts:

- Calories 92
- Fat: 1g
- Carbs: 15g
- Protein: 3g
- Sugar: 9g

10.7 Blueberries with lemon cream

- Preparation time: 5 minutes
- Cooking time: 0 minutes
- Serving: 6

Ingredients

- 1 cup vanilla yogurt, low-fat
- 8-ounce jar whipped topping, fat-free
- 3 tablespoons of lemon juice
- 2 teaspoons of lemon zest
- 1 1/2 cups (unsweetened) blueberries, frozen and thawed

Directions

- In a medium bowl, combine the yogurt, lemon zest, juice, and whipped topping.

- Give each dessert bowl a half-cup of the ingredients. Add 1/3 cup of blueberries on top and serve.

Nutritional facts:

- Calories 121
- Fat: 1g
- Carbs: 24g
- Protein: 2g
- Sugar: 14g

10.8 Peach–berry parfait

- Preparation time: 7 minutes
- Cooking time: 0 minutes
- Serving: 4

Ingredients

- A 0.3-ounce packet of mixed-berry gelatin, sugar-free
- 1 cup blueberries or raspberries, unsweetened
- 1 cup (unsweetened) peach slices
- 1/2 cup vanilla yogurt, low-fat
- 1 cup of water

Directions

- In a little saucepan over high heat, bring the water to a boil.
- In a medium bowl, combine the dry gelatin with the boiling water. Stir the mixture to combine the ingredients.
- When the mixture is cold, whisk in the frozen peaches. Just blend the berries in by gently folding them in.
- Place a quarter cup of fruited gelatin in each of the four parfait glasses. Add 1 spoonful of yogurt on top. Repeat the layers. Refrigerate for up to 24 hours, covered with plastic wrap, or chill until stiff, about 30 minutes.

Nutritional facts:

- Calories 75
- Fat: 1g
- Carbs: 15g
- Protein: 3g
- Sugar: 11g

10.9 Creamy berry mini tarts

- Preparation time: 5 minutes
- Cooking time: 0 minutes
- Serving: 7

Ingredients

- 1 cup berries, finely chopped
- 1/3 cup apricot all-fruit spread or prepared lemon curd
- 1 cup whipped topping, fat-free
- 15 shells mini-phyllo shells

Directions

- In a small glass bowl, place the fruit spread or lemon curd. Microwave for 20 seconds on HIGH or until just melted.
- Spoon 1 teaspoon of the smoothed-out mixture into each shell. Add 1 spoonful of fruit and 1 tablespoon of whipped cream to each...

Nutritional facts:

- Calories 149
- Fat: 3g
- Carbs: 27g

CHAPTER 11: SMOOTHIE AND DRINKS

11.1 Green smoothie

- o Preparation time: 10 minutes
- o Cooking time: 0 minutes
- o Serving: 1

Ingredients

- o ¼ avocado
- o 1 (large) banana
- o 1 cup (vanilla) almond milk, unsweetened
- o 1 cup baby kale, coarsely chopped
- o 1 tablespoon of chia seeds
- o 1 cup of ice cubes
- o 2 teaspoons of honey

Directions

- o In a blender, combine the almond milk, kale, chia
  seeds, banana, avocado, and honey. Blend at high speed until smooth and creamy. Blend in the ice till smooth.

Nutritional facts:

- o Calories 343
- o Fat: 6g
- o Carbs: 54g
- o Protein: 28g
- o Sugar: 28g

11.2 Pineapple strawberry smoothie

- o Preparation time: 5 minutes
- o Cooking time: 0 minutes
- o Serving: 1

Ingredients

- o 1 cup pineapple, chopped fresh
- o 1 cup strawberries, frozen
- o 1 tablespoon of almond butter
- o ¾ cup almond milk, + more if required

Directions

- o In a blender, combine almond milk, almond
  butter, strawberries, and pineapple. Process until smooth, adjusting the consistency with additional almond milk as necessary. Serve right away.

Nutritional facts:

- o Calories 255
- o Fat: 6g
- o Carbs: 39g
- o Protein: 28g
- o Sugar: 24g

11.4 Spinach smoothie

- o Preparation time: 5 minutes
- o Cooking time: 0 minutes
- o Serving: 2

Ingredients

- o ½ cup Greek yogurt
- o 2 tablespoons nut butter of choice
- o ¼ cup almond milk
- o ½ avocado pitted
- o 1 teaspoon of vanilla extract
- o 2 cups spinach

- o 1 cup of ice
- o Some drops of sweetener to taste

Directions

- o To a blender, add all the ingredients minus the ice. And blend it until smooth.
- o The ice should be added and pulsed until mostly pulverized.
- o The mixture should be smooth and creamy after blending.

Nutritional facts:

- o Calories 236
- o Fat: 16g
- o Carbs: 11g
- o Protein: 4g
- o Sugar: 11g

11.6 Leafy greens avocado smoothie

- o Preparation time: 10 minutes
- o Cooking time: 0 minutes
- o Serving: 2

Ingredients

- o 1 cup (baby) kale
- o 2 cups of baby spinach
- o 1 avocado
- o 2 mint sprigs
- o 2 cups of water
- o 1 tablespoon of lemon juice, freshly squeezed
- o ½ cup of ice cubes

Directions

- o The powerful blender should be filled with mint, kale, lemon juice, spinach, avocado, and water. Lastly, add the ice cubes.
- o Blend the ingredients at high speed until it is smooth.
- o You can add some drops of Stevia to the smoothie if you want it to be sweeter.

Nutritional facts:

- o Calories 186
- o Fat: 14g
- o Carbs: 12g
- o Protein: 3g
- o Sugar: 1.5g

11.8 Almond mango smoothie bowl

- o Preparation time: 10 minutes
- o Cooking time: 0 minutes
- o Serving: 2

Ingredients

- o ¼ cup banana, sliced
- o ½ cup mango, chopped
- o ¼ cup almond milk, unsweetened
- o ½ cup Greek yogurt, nonfat
- o 5 tablespoons (unsalted) almonds, divided
- o ⅛ teaspoon allspice, ground
- o ½ teaspoon of honey
- o ¼ cup of raspberries

Directions

- o Mango, banana, almond milk, yogurt, 3 tbsp of almonds, and allspice should all be thoroughly blended in a blender.

o Place the smoothie in a bowl and garnish with raspberries, the leftover 2 tbsp of almonds, and honey.

Nutritional facts:

o Calories 457

o Fat: 24g

o Carbs: 12g

o Protein: 21g

o Sugar: 29g

11.10 Carrot smoothie

o Preparation time: 10 minutes

o Cooking time: 15 minutes

o Serving: 3

Ingredients

o 1 cup carrots, sliced

o 1 ½ cups of ice cubes

o 1 cup of orange juice

o 3 pieces (1 inch) orange-peel curls

o ½ teaspoon orange peel, finely shredded

Directions

o Carrots should be cooked for about 15 minutes, or until extremely soft, in a small covered pot with a tiny amount of boiling water. Good drainage. Cool.

o Blend some carrots that have been drained. Orange juice and the finely minced orange peel should be added. Blend under cover until smooth. Ice cubes should be added; cover and blend till smooth. Add liquid to glasses. Add orange peel curls as a garnish if you like.

Nutritional facts:

o Calories 55

o Fat: 8g

o Carbs: 13g

o Protein: 2g

o Sugar: 5g

11.11 Pineapple smoothie

o Preparation time: 10 minutes

o Cooking time: 0 minutes

o Serving: 2

Ingredients

o 1 cup canned pineapple, cubed

o ¼ cup of water

o ½ cup vanilla yogurt, nonfat

o 2 ice cubes, crushed

o ¼ cup orange-pineapple -juice concentrate

Directions

o Blend all ingredients in a blender until it is smooth and foamy. Serve right away.

Nutritional facts:

o Calories 55

o Fat: 8g

o Carbs: 13g

o Protein: 2g

o Sugar: 5g

11.14 Coconut, chia seed & spinach smoothie

o Preparation time: 5 minutes

o Cooking time: 0 minutes

o Serving: 1

Ingredients

o 2 tablespoons chia seeds

- o 1 1/4 cups of coconut milk
- o 1 scoop of vanilla protein powder
- o 1 cup spinach
- o 2 ice cubes

Directions

- o Blend all ingredients in a blender until it is smooth and foamy. Serve right away.

Nutritional facts:

- o Calories 266
- o Fat: 2g
- o Carbs: 5g
- o Protein: 4g
- o Sugar: 0.8g

11.17 Tomato smoothie

- o Preparation time: 5 minutes
- o Cooking time: 0 minutes
- o Serving: 1

Ingredients

- o 1/2 avocado
- o 2 cups of tomatoes
- o 1/4 cup of celery
- o 2 cups of ice
- o 1 tablespoon of lemon juice
- o 1/2 cup tomato juice, low-salt
- o a dash of salt
- o hot sauce to taste

Directions

- o Blend the ingredients until they are well combined. Try adding some water, beginning with 1/4 cup, if the smoothie is too thick.

Nutritional facts:

- o Calories 204
- o Fat: 13g
- o Carbs: 19g
- o Protein: 9g
- o Sugar: 3g

11.20 Hot cocoa

- o Preparation time: 10 minutes
- o Cooking time: 0 minutes
- o Serving: 12

Ingredients

- o 2-1/3 cups instant-dry milk, nonfat
- o 1/3 cup diabetic sugar
- o 1/3 cup cocoa, unsweetened
- o chocolate milk bar, shavings
- o candy (sugar-free) canes (optional)
- o milk (fat-free) frothed (optional)

Directions

- o In a big bowl, combine cocoa, dry milk, and sweetener; whisk thoroughly.
- o Stir 1/4 cup of cocoa mix into 1 cup of hot water in a mug to serve. Add frothed fat-free milk on top and top with chopped chocolate.
- o Keep any leftover cocoa mixture in an airtight container.

Nutritional facts:

- o Calories 62
- o Fat: 0.6g
- o Carbs: 14g
- o Protein: 5g
- o Sugar: 0.4g

60 DAYS MEAL PLAN

Day	Breakfast	Lunch	Dinner	Exercise
1	Scrambled eggs with spinach and raspberry	Thrice-bean balsamic salad	Cauliflower soup	30-minute walk
2	Fried veggies and eggs	Avocado-onion salad	Beef tenderloin	30-minute bike ride
3	Oatmeal with milk (overnight)	Chicken choppy salad	Southwest-style grilled steak with vibrant skillet veggies	20-minute squat
4	Power parfait	Watermelon-cucumber salad with mint	Simple meatballs	20-minute yoga
5	Yogurt pancakes	Asparagus spear lemony salad	Beef with sweet ginger sauce	30-minute swim
6	Rapidly cooked oats	Tomato artichoke toss	Sirloin hoagies	30-minute neck stretch
7	Breakfast bowl with quinoa	Creamy cucumber dill salad	Cumin-seasoned beef patties	Rest day
8	Mushroom-cheese omelet	Bean salsa salad	Chili-stuffed potatoes	20-minute yoga
9	Grilled rye and Swiss cheese	Tangy pepper-sweet carrot salad	Spicy sirloin steak	30-minute walk
10	Raisin toast with apricot spread	Crispy, crunchy coleslaw	Beef stewed and ale	30-minute hamstring stretch
11	French toast	Mustard-romaine salad	Steak fajitas	30-minute swim
12	Traditional avocado toast	1,000 island wedges	Tendered green pepper	20-minute yoga
13	Greek yogurt with nuts and fruits	Cumin and Picante salad	Spicy sirloin steak	30-minute jogging
14	Scrambled eggs with spinach and raspberry	Cauliflower soup	Pork chops	Rest day
15	Fried veggies and eggs	Mushroom soup with sherry	Pork with rice	30-minute swim
16	Oatmeal with milk (overnight)	Wild rice and turkey soup	Molasses drumsticks	20-minute yoga
17	Power parfait	Tomato and pepper soup	Lemon Greek chicken	30-minute walk
18	Yogurt pancakes	Very soup	Chicken lemon pasta	30-minute bike ride
19	Rapidly cooked oats	Green pepper soup	Barbecued peachy chicken	30-minute swim
20	Breakfast bowl with quinoa	Sweet corn and peppers soup	Taco-chicken tenders	20-minute yoga
21	Mushroom-cheese omelet	Green onion and cream potato soup	Rosemary Dijon chicken	Rest day

22	Grilled rye and Swiss cheese	Green peppers tilapia stew	Spinach and goat cheese stuffed chicken	30-minute bike ride
23	Raisin toast with apricot spread	Minestrone soup	Lemony au jus chicken	30-minute swim
24	French toast	Potato soup	Crispy chicken in a hot chipotle cream sauce	20-minute yoga
25	Traditional avocado toast	Rutabaga stew	White-wine mushroom chicken	30-minute walk
26	Greek yogurt with nuts and fruits	Mango Gazpacho	Tangy chicken and peppers	30-minute dancing
27	Scrambled eggs with spinach and raspberry	Garlic aioli tuna steaks	Hoisin chicken	Rest day
28	Fried veggies and eggs	Walnut tomato tilapia	Skillet chicken	30-minutes of brisk walking
29	Rosemary walnuts	Walnut tomato tilapia	Cauliflower soup	30-minutes of jogging or running
30	Raisin toast with apricot spread	Thrice-bean balsamic salad	Beef tenderloin	20-minutes of balance exercises
31	French toast	Avocado-onion salad	Southwest-style grilled steak with vibrant skillet veggies	30-minutes of aerobics
32	Traditional avocado toast	Chicken choppy salad	Simple meatballs	20-minutes of jump rope
33	Greek yogurt with nuts and fruits	Watermelon-cucumber salad with mint	Beef with sweet ginger sauce	20-minutes of kettlebell exercises
34	Scrambled eggs with spinach and raspberry	Asparagus spear lemony salad	Rosemary cheesy kale chips	30-minute swim
35	Fried veggies and eggs	Tomato artichoke toss	Air-fry radishes	Rest day
36	Rosemary walnuts	Creamy cucumber dill salad	Lemon and herb cauliflower (Air-fryer)	30-minute walk
37	Yogurt pancakes	Crispy, crunchy coleslaw	Homemade guacamole	30-minute bike ride
38	Rapidly cooked oats	Mustard-romaine salad	Sweet peanut buttery dip	20-minutes lunge
39	Breakfast bowl with quinoa	1,000 island wedges	Marinated mushrooms	20-minutes Hamstring stretch
40	Mushroom-cheese omelet	Cumin and Picante salad	Cumin-seasoned beef patties	20-minutes shoulder stretch
41	Grilled rye and Swiss cheese	Cauliflower soup	Chili-stuffed potatoes	20 minutes of bodyweight exercises
42	Marinated mushrooms	Mushroom soup with sherry	Onion roast	Rest day
43	Rosemary walnuts	Wild rice and turkey soup	Beef stewed and ale	30-minutes of brisk walking

44	Lemony shrimp	Tomato and pepper soup	Steak fajitas	30-minute bike ride
45	Lime blueberries	Very soup	Tendered green pepper	30-minute swim
46	Carrots with spicy cream dip	Mango Gazpacho	Spicy sirloin steak	20-minute yoga
47	Fried veggies and eggs	Garlic aioli tuna steaks	Pork chops	30-minute walk
48	Rosemary walnuts	Walnut tomato tilapia	Pork with rice	30-minute bike ride
49	Raisin toast with apricot spread	Walnut tomato tilapia	Molasses drumsticks	Rest day
50	French toast	Thrice-bean balsamic salad	Lemon Greek chicken	20 –minutes squats
51	Traditional avocado toast	Avocado-onion salad	Skillet chicken	20-minutes push-ups
52	Traditional avocado toast	Chicken choppy salad	Cauliflower soup	30-minute swim
53	Greek yogurt with nuts and fruits	Watermelon-cucumber salad with mint	Beef tenderloin	20-minute yoga
54	Scrambled eggs with spinach and raspberry	Asparagus spear lemony salad	Southwest-style grilled steak with vibrant skillet veggies	30-minute jogging
55	Fried veggies and eggs	Tomato artichoke toss	Simple meatballs	30-minute bike ride
56	Oatmeal with milk (overnight)	Avocado-onion salad	Beef with sweet ginger sauce	Rest day
57	Power parfait	Chicken choppy salad	Lemon Greek chicken	20-minute yoga
58	Yogurt pancakes	Watermelon-cucumber salad with mint	Chicken lemon pasta	30-minute walk
59	Rapidly cooked oats	Asparagus spear lemony salad	Barbecued peachy chicken	30-minute bike ride
60	Breakfast bowl with quinoa	Tomato artichoke toss	Taco-chicken tenders	Rest day

DIABETES JOURNAL

(PRINTED VERSION)

	1	2	3	4	5	6	7	8	9	10	11	12	13	14	15	16	17	18	19	20	21	22	23	24	25	26	27	28	29	30	31
awakening																															
insulin																															
2h after breakfast																															
before lunch																															
insulin																															
2h after lunch																															
before dinner																															
insulin																															
2h after dinner																															
before bedtime																															
insulin																															
at night																															

GET YOUR BONUSES NOW

Diabetes Journal (Digital version) - Healing Diabetes through Exercise - Easy Pre-Diabetes Cookbook for Better Health - Diabetic Air Fryer Cookbook - Foods Lists for Diabetes

OR

[CLICK HERE](#)

CONCLUSION

The "Diabetic Cookbook for the Newly Diagnosed" is a thorough and helpful resource for people who have just received a diabetes diagnosis. It provides practical advice and insights on managing the condition through dietary changes, making it an essential resource.

This cookbook stands out for its emphasis on healthy and delicious recipes that cater to the dietary needs of people with diabetes. It offers a diverse selection of recipes that provide balanced nutrition and are enjoyable to eat, making it easy for readers to find dishes they will love.

In addition to recipes, the book offers guidance on monitoring blood sugar levels, selecting healthy foods, and controlling portion sizes. These are critical factors in effectively managing diabetes and reducing the risk of complications.

Additionally, the "Diabetic Cookbook for the Newly Diagnosed" is written in straightforward language that anyone may understand, regardless of their level of diabetes understanding. The book is a great resource for individuals who are unfamiliar with the condition because the author takes the time to explain the science behind the illness, including how it affects the body and the function of insulin.

The book provides a wealth of knowledge on controlling diabetes through dietary changes, including scrumptious and healthful recipes, suggestions for controlling blood sugar levels, and explanations of the science behind the condition. Anyone wishing to take control of their health and efficiently manage their diabetes should read it.

REFERENCES

https://diabetes.org/diabetes/newly-diagnosed

https://healthlibrary.askapollo.com/4-common-diabetes-related-fears-people-have-and-how-to-overcome-them/

https://www.medicalnewstoday.com/articles/318472#Key-facts-about-diabetes-in-the-US

https://dtc.ucsf.edu/newly-diagnosed/

https://medlineplus.gov/ency/patientinstructions/000964.htm

https://www.mayoclinic.org/diseases-conditions/type-2-diabetes/symptoms-causes/syc-20351193

https://www.webmd.com/diabetes/type-2-diabetes

https://kidshealth.org/en/parents/type2.html

https://www.healthline.com/health/type-2-diabetes/treatment-newly-diagnosed

https://www.niddk.nih.gov/health-information/diabetes/overview/diet-eating-physical-activity

https://www.dietdoctor.com/diabetes/diet#diabetes-diet

https://www.medicalnewstoday.com/articles/317355#foods-for-other-conditions

https://www.cdc.gov/diabetes/managing/eat-well/meal-plan-method.html

https://www.dietdoctor.com/diabetes/diet#diabetes-diet

https://www.allrecipes.com/recipe/259711/overnight-oatmeal-with-milk/

https://www.allrecipes.com/recipe/257457/meyer-lemon-avocado-toast/

https://www.allrecipes.com/recipe/256156/overnight-light-pbj-oats/

https://www.tasteofhome.com/recipes/yogurt-pancakes/

https://www.tasteofhome.com/recipes/minty-watermelon-cucumber-salad/

https://www.thediabetescouncil.com/6-easy-salad-recipes-to-help-control-diabetes/

https://www.tasteofhome.com/collection/diabetic-friendly-potluck-salads/

https://www.tasteofhome.com/recipes/no-fuss-avocado-onion-salad/

https://www.allrecipes.com/recipe/235307/classic-turkey-and-rice-soup

https://www.eatingwell.com/recipes/22881/health-condition/diabetic/soups/

https://www.allrecipes.com/recipes/1700/healthy-recipes/diabetic/soups-and-stews/

https://www.tasteofhome.com/collection/diabetic-soups/

https://www.tasteofhome.com/recipes/air-fryer-steak-fajitas/

https://www.eatingwell.com/gallery/7989033/diabetes-friendly-air-fryer-recipes/

https://diabeticgourmet.com/diabetic-recipe/grilled-southwestern-steak-and-colorful-skillet-vegetables

https://www.tasteofhome.com/collection/diabetic-beef-recipes/

https://www.thediabetescouncil.com/12-meat-recipes-for-people-with-diabetes/

https://www.tasteofhome.com/collection/quick-diabetic-friendly-chicken-dinners/

https://www.eatingwell.com/recipe/250833/white-turkey-chili/

https://www.diabeticfoodie.com/10-easy-diabetic-chicken-recipes/

https://www.eatingwell.com/gallery/7989033/diabetes-friendly-air-fryer-recipes/?slide=7b6d1c02-c181-42d1-9cff-0c4ec67bf4c8#7b6d1c02-c181-42d1-9cff-0c4ec67bf4c8

https://www.tasteofhome.com/collection/diabetic-snacks/

https://www.allrecipes.com/recipe/270825/air-fryer-plantain-chips/

https://www.eatingwell.com/recipes/18350/health-condition/diabetic/side-dishes/

https://www.tasteofhome.com/collection/diabetic-side-dishes/

https://www.tasteofhome.com/collection/diabetic-fish-seafood-recipes/

https://www.eatingwell.com/recipes/19955/health-condition/diabetic/dinner/fish-seafood/

https://diabeticgourmet.com/recipes/diabetic-seafood-recipes

https://diabetesstrong.com/10-healthy-low-carb-seafood-recipes/

https://www.everydaydiabeticrecipes.com/FishandSeafood

https://www.eatingwell.com/recipes/18355/health-condition/diabetic/desserts/

https://diabetesstrong.com/easy-diabetic-desserts/

https://www.tasteofhome.com/collection/diabetic-desserts/

https://www.allrecipes.com/recipes/1692/healthy-recipes/diabetic/desserts/

https://www.eatingwell.com/recipes/19948/health-condition/diabetic/drinks/smoothies/

https://www.healthline.com/health/diabetes/diabetic-friendly-smoothies

https://www.diabeticfoodie.com/smoothies/

https://www.eatingwell.com/recipes/18342/health-condition/diabetic/drinks/

https://www.verywellhealth.com/type-2-diabetes-nutrition-and-weight-loss-4014311

https://www.verywellfit.com/can-you-prevent-diabetes-with-diet-and-exercise-5195526

https://www.heart.org/en/health-topics/diabetes/prevention--treatment-of-diabetes/the-diabetic-diet

MEASUREMENT CONVERSION CHART

Temperature Conversions:

Celsius	Fahrenheit
0°C	32°F
100°C	212°F
150°C	302°F
180°C	356°F
200°C	392°F
220°C	428°F
250°C	482°F

Weight Conversions:

Metric	Imperial	US Customary
1 gram	0.035 oz.	0.04 oz.
100 grams	3.5 oz.	3.5 oz.
250 grams	8.8 oz.	8.8 oz.
500 grams	1.1 lb.	1.1 lb.
1 kg	2.2 lb.	2.2 lb.

Volume Conversions:

Metric	Imperial	US Customary
1 ml	0.03 FL oz.	0.03 FL oz.
100 ml	3.4 FL oz.	3.4 FL oz.
250 ml	8.5 FL oz.	8.5 FL oz.
500 ml	17 FL oz.	2.1 cups
1 liter	1.8 pints	4.2 cups

NOTES

Made in United States
North Haven, CT
18 October 2023

42897771R00052